AF292704

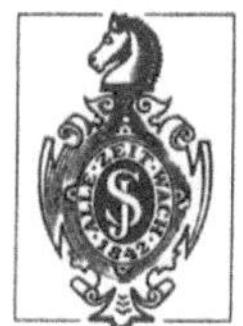

Knut Holtedahl

Early Diagnosis of Cancer in General Practice

A Manual

Springer-Verlag
Berlin Heidelberg New York
London Paris Tokyo Hong Kong

Dr. Knut Holtedahl
Balsfjordgt 32
N-9000 Tromsø

ISBN-13: 978-3-540-51252-3   e-ISBN-13: 978-3-642-74816-5
DOI: 10.1007/ 978-3-642-74816-5

Library of Congress Cataloging-in-Publication Data
Holtedahl, Knut. Early diagnosis of cancer in general practice: a manual / Knut
Holtedahl. p. cm. Includes bibliographical references.

1. Cancer-Diagnosis.   2. Family medicine.   I. Title.

The use of registered names, trademarks, etc. in this publication does not imply,
even in the absence of a specific statement, that names are exempt from the relevant
protective laws and regulations and therefore free for general use.

Product liability: The publisher can give no guarantee for information about drug
dosage and application thereof contained in this book, in every individual case the
respective user must check its accuracy by consulting other pharmaceutical
literature.

Typesetting: Hagedorn, Berlin; Printing: Langenscheidt, Berlin;

2119/3020-543210 – Printed on acid-free paper.

Preface

I had not been practising medicine for long before I was blaming myself for unnecessarily delayed diagnoses of cancer in some of my patients. Looking back, I thought I could have put more knowledge, effort and understanding into some of the consultations. I soon started to collect and organize information, drawing on the literature as well as on my regular work in general practice. Colleagues have helped me adjust my ideas to reality when I have participated in teaching about cancer on courses for general practitioners.

This book is the product of these labours. I hope it will find a place on the general practitioner's desktop or on the nearest bookshelf, inviting frequent use as a quick source of reference. Specialists too may find it useful for reminders, and so may medical students.

The Norwegian Cancer Society has been a generous supporter of my research about cancer in general practice, including the work for this book. The earliest stages of the research work were also supported by the Norwegian Medical Association. The Cancer Registry of Norway has on several occasions furnished necessary information. The frequency tables in Part 3 have been kindly furnished by the cancer registries for Scotland, England and Wales, Canada and the State of Iowa, USA. Several colleagues in different departments at the University Hospital of Tromsø, Norway, have given valuable positive criticism of drafts.

Tromsø, December 1989   Knut Holtedahl

Contents

Introduction

The Challenge: Avoiding Diagnostic Delay

In 15 years of general practice I have had many opportunities to witness the course of cancer in a patient. The question "Was the diagnosis made as early as possible?" is almost always important to the patient as well as to the doctor. Although the topic is complex and proof is often difficult, early diagnosis is favoured in most cases of cancer [1]. Pack and Gallo [2], 50 years ago, made the first modern study of "patient delay" and "doctor delay" in cancer treatment. Many later studies, including my own [3], have concluded as they did: the time from the first symptom until diagnosis is unreasonably long for a great number of cancer patients.

The population of any general practice is usually typical of the ordinary population in the community. In such a population most general practitioners will see no more than one case of breast or colorectal cancer every year. The total number of new cases of cancer in general practice rarely exceeds ten per year. On the other hand, *excluding* cancer is daily work. Nylenna and Bruusgaard [4] found that 13.2% of all encounters in general practice dealt with patients expressing fear of cancer, having a known malignancy or being further investigated for a cancer-related reason. Norwegian general practitioners recorded one or more of the seven warning signals of cancer in 5,4% of encounters, or in approximately 1 out of every 20 patients [5]. Such signals are published by cancer associations in most countries in order to make the public aware of early symptoms and to encourage them to see a doctor should they experience one. The dilemma of general practitioners as well as of most people is in distinguishing evil from nuisance. For example, indigestion may be a symptom of cancer, but it is also present in most gastrointestinal disorders, which in Norway in 1978 accounted for 5,7% of the total number of diagnoses in general practice [6].

A simple solution does not exist. This manual proposes routines and methods of reasoning which may increase the efficiency of cancer diagnostic work in general practice, without encouraging unnecessary procedures.

Using the Manual

Red Flags: Initiating the Diagnostic Process

Williams [7] emphasizes the importance of looking for clues or "red flags" in general practice. Such clues may be essential in order to form correct diagnostic hypotheses, the starting point of most diagnostic work in general practice [8]. Seven warning signals have been selected for public health education purposes, but they also serve as reminders for doctors. General practitioners should be able to use a much more refined set of clues when considering cancer. Such clues may refer to personal characteristics, previous or chronic diseases, or to the course of the present disease. Symptoms like the warning signals may serve as clues, but the general practitioner should be able to give an immediate anatomical context to each symptom. With the benefit of medical knowledge, symptoms may be more refined clues for a doctor than for a layman.

Finally, awareness of diagnostic pitfalls is important. Some of these are general, others are specific to cancer diagnostics. The general practitioner should routinely check promising diagnostic hypotheses against such traps. The first section of this manual summarizes data clues, symtom clues and diagnostic traps.

Organ Systems: Thinking Anatomy

During the diagnostic process it is important to visualize the anatomy relevant to the hypotheses. The second section of the manual is divided into anatomic subgroups corresponding to organ systems defined by the Norwegian Cancer Registry. The subgroup "Other and unspecified sites" has been subdivided in this manual into skin, eye, central nervous system, thyroid, and bone/muscles/connective tissue.

Every organ system has been divided into single organs or anatomic sites. *Common symptoms, diagnostic clues* and recommendations for *follow-up* are described for each site. The information and evaluation have been kept brief, necessitating some compromise as to precision and completeness. The manual does not give detailed procedures for routine consultations; it is chiefly intended as a useful source of reference when the doctor feels uncertain, when a symptom or a constellation of symptoms is unusual or persists longer than expected, or when the patient belongs to a risk group for some form of cancer.

Diagnostic clues are grouped according to elements in the diagnostic process: knowledge of epidemiology or anatomo-pathology, medical history, clinical examination, and supplementary tests and examinations performed or ordered during the encounter. Risk factors are described under the heading "Epidemiology" rather than under "Medical History". General practitioners often have previous knowledge of such risk factors in their patients, but if not, active questioning is necessary. Some obvious points have not been repeated for each organ; for instance that the taking of the medical history, the clinical examination and the initial ordering of blood tests should be related to the presenting symptom and to any other factors revealed during the encounter; that haemoglobin concentrations and sedimentation rates should be widely used (their measurement is proposed separately only exceptionally); and that, for most organs, the risk of cancer increases with age. It is most of all in regard to older people that general practitioners should lower their "cancer suspicion threshold". It has been shown that, in view of the incidence rates, general practitioners have an irrationally lower threshold for suspecting cancer in females than in males, and in younger people than in old [9].

Follow-up may be performed in the general practitioner's own consulting room or by referral. Some examinations which are commonly ordered although not performed by general practitioners are listed under "Supplementary Tests and Examinations".

Frequency Tables and Diagnostic Indexes: Thinking Probabilities

General practitioners should not be afraid of a quantitative approach to diagnostic thinking. The low prevalence of almost any important disease in most general practice populations certainly constitutes a handicap for general practitioners compared to hospital doctors who work with selected populations. On the other hand, where is a hospital doctor would require a 90% probability of disease in order to start treatment with potent drugs, disease probabilities of 10% – 15% at the end an encounter may be sufficient in general practice. With important diseases like cancer, the search should sometimes be continued at even lower levels of probability, either by referral to a specialist or by a later follow-up appointment.

As a basis for such estimates, the ten most frequent forms of cancer for both sexes in the UK and parts of North America are presented in Part 3 of the manual. Tables for different age groups are also presented.

Some tables will be found integrated in the text in Part 2. These tables present sex- and age-distributed calculations of diagnostic indexes for some important cancer symptoms in relation to some major forms of cancer. They are based on a Norwegian study of cancer patients [10, 11] and on the warning signal recordings in general practice [5]. The indexes are *positive predictive value* (the frequency of disease among the patients presenting the symptom) and *likelihood ratio* (the proportion of the diseased who experience the symptom divided by the proportion of the non-diseased who experience the symptom) [12]. Such calculations are desirable because encounters in general practice usually start with some kind of symptom presentation. Subsequent diagnostic hypotheses need to be examined in relation to these symptoms. Calculations are possible according to Bayes' formula if there is access to three probability estimates: the probability of cancer $P(C)$, which corresponds to the prevalence in the population of the general practice; the probability of the symptom $P(S)$

in the same population; and the sensitivity − the probability that the symptom indicates cancer − at the time of the encounter, $P(S \mid C)$.

Cancer incidence rates do not differ very much between Western countries, and extrapolation of the diagnostic indexes to other settings may seem tempting. However, the propensity of patients to present symptoms in general practice may vary with time and from place to place, as may the prevalence of cancer in general practice encounters. The tables therefore present probability tendencies rather than definite percentages and ratios. The main value of the tables is that they show the variation in probability at different ages and for each sex, as well as the difference in approximate probability levels between different symptoms and different forms of cancer. Also, low probabilities remind us that single symptoms may be a good starting point, but rarely furnish a sufficient basis for decisions. Sound decisions must be based on a combination of selected pieces of diagnostic information.

The indexes have been replaced by a dash (−) when background data are insufficient. A detailed discussion of background statistics and estimates has been presented elsewhere [13, 14].

For colorectal cancer, a revision of probabilities has been made based on the results of tests for occult blood in stools of patients presenting with "Indigestion or changes in bowel habits which have not rapidly normalized". A similar probability revision is shown for lung cancer in patients who cough, according to whether or not they are daily smokers [15]. Again the numeric values should be interpreted with caution because prior probabilities are not necessarily the same everywhere, but the tables are of value in illustrating the difference between prior and posterior probabilities. The difference in many cases is important enough to have practical consequences.

I would like to add that the diagnostic challenge offered by the more rare forms of cancer can be met only by being mentally prepared that sooner or later one or two such cancers will appear in every practice. This is also a matter of probability; there are many rare forms, and together they constitute an important group of cancers. This manual should demonstrate that rare cancers — as well as common cancers occurring in age groups where they are uncommon — are not necessarily the most difficult to diagnose if they are thought of.

Finally, flow charts suggesting follow-up of a low haemoglobin concentration or a high sedimentation rate are included in Part 3.

References

1. Holtedahl KA, Rosengren B (1985) Almenpraktikerens rolle i tidlig-diagnostikk av kreft (The role of the general practitioner in the early diagnosis of cancer). In: Nylenna M, Gundersen S, Johannessen JV (eds) Kreft i almenpraksis. Universitetsforlaget, Oslo
2. Pack GT, Gallo JS (1938) The culpability for delay in the treatment of cancer. Am J Cancer 33: 443–462
3. Holtedahl KA (1980) Kreftdiagnostikk i almenpraksis I (Diagnosis of cancer in general practice I. Can the diagnosis be made earlier?). Tidsskr Nor Laegeforen 100: 1219–1226 (English summary)
4. Nylenna M, Bruusgaard D (1986) Dimensions of the cancer problem in general practice. Allgemeinmedizin 15: 85–93
5. Holtedahl KA (1984) Kreftdiagnostikk i almenpraksis III (Diagnosis of cancer in general practice III. General practitioners' recording of the seven warning signals of cancer in patients). Tidsskr Nor Laegeforen 104: 799–807 (English summary)
6. Rutle O (1983) Pasienten fram i lyset (Throwing light on the patient). Thesis. National Institute of Public Health, Health Services Research Unit, Oslo (Report No. 3, with English summary)
7. Williams T (1977) A strategy for defining the clinical content of family medicine. J Fam Pract 4: 497–499
8. Barrows HS, Norman GR, Neufeld VR, Feightner JW (1982) The clinical reasoning of randomly selected physicians in general medical practice. Clin Invest Med 5: 49–55
9. Nylenna M (1986) Diagnosis cancer in general practice: When is cancer suspected? Br Med J 293: 245–248
10. Holtedahl KA (1984) Kreftdiagnostikk i almenpraksis V (Diagnosis of cancer in general practice V. Patients with and without cancer). Tidsskr Nor Laegeforen 104: 804–806 (English summary)
11. Holtedahl KA (1987) The value of warning signals of cancer in general practice. Scand J Prim Health Care 5: 140–143
12. Weinstein MC, Fineberg HV (1980) Clinical decision analysis. Saunders, Philadelphia
13. Holtedahl KA. A method of calculating diagnostic indexes for possible cancer symptoms in general practice. Accepted for publication in Allgemeinmedizin, 1990
14. Holtedahl KA. More diagnostic indexes from general practice for some important forms of cancer. Accepted for publication in Allgemeinmedizin, 1990
15. Holtedahl KA. Probability revision in general practice: the cases of occult blood in stool in patients with indigestion, and daily smoking in patients who cough. Accepted for publication in Allgemeinmedizin, 1990

Part 1.
Red Flags

Early Clues To Cancer

Data Clues

Clues Related to Personal Characteristics

(Age, habits, body size, skin colour, parity, sexual practice, family, profession and social class)

Increased risk of cancer	Most relevant organ or form of cancer
Increasing age	
Smoking	Bronchi
	Larynx
	Lip
	Oral cavity
	Bladder
	Pancreas
	Oesophagus
	Cervix uteri
High intake of alcohol	Oesophagus
	Larynx
	Oral cavity
	Mamma
	Liver
	Pancreas
	Sigmoid colon
Intravenous drug abuse	Various cancers secondary to human immunodeficiency virus (HIV) infection, especially lymphoma
Low intake of vegetables	Gastrointestinal cancers
	Bronchi
Proneness to sunburn	Skin
No children or low parity	Mamma
	Corpus uteri
	Ovary
Early menarche, late menopause and high age at last birth, except if high parity	Mamma
	Corpus uteri

Table continued

Table continued from page 13

Increased risk of cancer	Most relevant organ or form of cancer
Large body surface (height/weight)	Mamma in postmenopausal women Corpus uteri
Low age at first birth	Cervix uteri
Many sexual partners	Cervix uteri. Indirect risk of other cancers secondary to HIV infection
Male homosexuality	Kaposi's sarcoma and other cancers secondary to HIV infection
Cancer in close family members	Especially colon (polyposis), but different organ locations possible in one family. Uterus, breast, stomach are not uncommon sites. Members of "cancer families" involving two or more generations have an increased risk of cancer at a relatively young age, and of multiple cancers
Workers exposed to dust or chemicals	Bladder Bronchi Nose Liver Leukaemia
Low socioeconomic class	Cervix uteri Stomach Rectum Bronchi Bladder

Clues Related to Previous, Chronic or Present Disease

Increased risk of cancer	Most relevant organ or form of cancer
Previous cancer	
HIV infection	Kaposi's sarcoma, lymphoma (see above)
Former gastrectomy	Stump cancer
Anacidity	Stomach
Coeliac disease	Lymphoma of small intestine
Ulcerative colitis	Colon
Hypertonia	Kidney
Gallstones/former cholecystitis	Gall bladder. In younger women also breast, internal genitalia, gastrointestinal tract
Previous or ongoing immunosuppressive therapy, for instance after kidney transplantation	
Down's syndrome	Leukaemia
Progression of present symptoms	

Symptom Clues

Symptom	Most relevant organ	More specific description of symptoms
Sore	Skin	
	Mucous membranes	
	Mouth	
	Nose	
	Ear	
	Genital organs	
Lump	Breast	
	Neck	
	Axilla	
	Groin	
	Bone	
	Muscle	
Pain	Sinus	
	Stomach	Epigastric pain
	Pancreas	Vague but constant pain
	Kidney	
	Bone (especially long bones and vertebrae)	
	Central nervous system	Headache
		Backache especially when lying on the back: spinal cord, but vertebrae, pancreas, kidney as well
Stenosis, irritation	Sinus	Nasal stenosis
	Larynx	Hoarseness
	Bronchi	Cough, dyspnoea, infection
	Oesophagus	Difficulty in swallowing
	Biliary tract	Icterus
	Cerebellopontine angle	Unilateral loss of hearing, noise in the ear, dizziness
	Pituitary	Unilateral loss of vision, sometimes endocrine symptoms
	Spinal cord	Pain usually precedes loss of sensibility
		Paresis sometimes early sign

Table continued

Table continued from page 16

Symptom	Most relevant organ	More specific description of symptoms
	Cerebrum	Nausea/vomiting, dizziness, mental changes, epilepsy
Bleeding (macroscopic/ microscopic/ cutaneous)	Epipharynx/nose Bronchi Stomach Colon Uterus/vagina Kidney Bladder Prostate Skin (leukaemia)	
General symptoms	Stomach	Nausea, weight loss, weakness
	Pancreas	Weight loss
	Kidney	Weight loss, weakness
	Central nervous system	Nausea, vomiting. dizziness
	Lymphoma	Weakness, moderate fever
	Leukaemia	Weakness, moderate fever
Paraneoplasias (Non-metastatic distant manifestations)		
Poly-neuritis	Most often lung	Sensibility/reflexes diminished, sometimes paresis
Endocrino-pathy	Most often lung	ACTH (Cushing's) syndrome
	Most often mamma	Hypercalcaemia, renal calculus
	Pancreas	Gastrinoma/stomach ulcer
Cutaneous	Most often lymphomas/ myelomas/leukaemias or adenocarcinomas	Acanthosis nigrans (axilla) Acquired ichthyosis Generalized pruritus Erythrodermia Purpura Dermatomyositis (face/eyelids: erythema, oedema, telangiectases) Repeated attacks of thrombophlebitis

ACTH, adrenocorticotropic hormone

Symptom clues necessitate: 1. Examination
2. Evaluation
3. Control if the conclusion remains uncertain

Diagnostic Traps

When early cancer seems possible, remember:

1. *Negative results of examinations do not exclude cancer.* These include laboratory tests, X-ray examinations and clinical examinations.
2. *Positive tests must be verified and followed up.* Writing them down in the medical record is not enough.
3. *Diagnosis of any common disease does not exclude simultaneous cancer.*
4. *Increasing incidence with increasing age does not exclude cancer in younger persons.*
5. *Former traumas may or may not be responsible for new symptoms.* The quickest explanation of symptoms is not always the right one.
6. *Vague symptoms sometimes may become less vague with the help of a good medical history.* Chronology, location, intensity, progression should be considered.
7. *Confusing symptoms may reveal (or hide) endocrine disorders, while endocrine disorders may reveal (or hide) a tumour.*

Part 2.
Organ Systems and
Individual Anatomic Sites

Lip

Common Symptoms

A sore which does not heal

Diagnostic Clues

Clinical Examination

Usually lower lip

Anatomopathology

Usually spindle cell carcinomas

Follow-up

By the General Practitioner

If sore present < 1 month

By Referral to Specialist

If sore present > 1 month: otorhinolaryngologist, dermatologist or surgeon

Tongue

Common Symptoms

A sore, a lump or a wart

Lymphadenopathy may be presenting symptom

Diagnostic Clues

Clinical Examination

Inspection of dorsal part of tongue using tongue depressor

Bidigital palpation

Follow-up

By Referral to Specialist

Otorhinolaryngologist as soon as possible

Salivary Glands

Common Symptoms

A lump

An intraoral swelling

Pain/paresis of facial nerve possible if growth is rapid

Diagnostic Clues

Epidemiology

Location of salivary gland tumours:

80% in the parotid gland
5%–10% in the submandibular gland
Various intraoral locations, most frequently in the palate
Tumour in the sublingual gland is rare

Approximately one of four or five salivary gland tumours is malignant, but the malignancy fraction varies for different locations. For the submandibular gland and for the salivary gland tumours in the palate the ratio benign:malignant is about 1:1, for the parotid gland 5–7:1

Clinical Examination

Palpation usually cannot distinguish benign tumours (and sometimes even inflammations) from cancers

Most parotid tumours arise in the superficial lobe, mostly with an infra-auricular, retromandibular location. A more ventral location in the cheek may occur when the tumour arises in accessory salivary gland tissue close to the parotid excretory duct

Follow-up

By Referral to Specialist

Any salivary gland swelling which is not acute viral parotitis: otorhinolaryngologist

Gums/Buccal Mucosa/Palate/Floor of Oral Cavity

Common Symptoms

Relatively innocent-looking mucosal lesion (sore/infiltration/ papilloma)

Leukoplakia may precede the above

A swelling

Diagnostic Clues

Epidemiology

Increased risk:　　All forms of tobacco use
　　　　　　　　　　High intake of alcohol

Incidence ratio males : females is approximately 2 : 1

Clinical Examination

Bidigital palpation

Palpation of collum

Anatomopathology

Palatine tumours usually arise either in the squamous epithelium of the mucous membrane or in accessory salivary gland tissue

Follow-up

By the General Practitioner

If lesion present < 1 month

By Referral to Specialist

Any leukoplakia

Other lesions which persist > 1 month: otorhinolaryngologist

Tonsils

Common Symptoms

A sore, a lump or a wart

Asymmetry

Lymphadenopathy may be presenting symptom

Follow-up

By Referral to Specialist

Otorhinolaryngologist

Nasopharynx

Common Symptoms

Unilateral loss of hearing

Unilateral ear pain

Unilateral noise in the ear

Nasal stenosis possible

Lymphadenopathy may be presenting symptom

Ear symptoms or nasal stenosis each occur in about three out of four patients before diagnosis

Diagnostic Clues

Clinical Examination

Inspection of palate: bulging?

Tympanic membrane freely moving? (Unilateral secretory otitis is a fairly common finding)

Palpation of collum

Anatomopathology

In the parapharyngeal spatium, limited laterally by the parotids, cranially by the base of the skull and caudally by the hyoid bone, approximately half of the tumours are salivary gland tumours, arising in the deep structures of the parotid or in ectopic tissue. Most of these are adenomas. Approximately one-third are benign neurogenic tumours and approximately one-fifth are malignant tumours

Follow-up

By the General Practitioner

If duration of symptoms < 1 month and clinical examination of ear/buccal cavity/pharynx/neck is negative

By Referral to Specialist

If duration of symptoms > 1 month or if there are positive clinical findings: otorhinolaryngologist

Hypopharynx

Common Symptoms

The sensation of a lump high up in the throat

Lymphadenopathy may be presenting symptom

Diagnostic Clues

Clinical Examination

Laryngoscopy (see Larynx) with inspection of the region oral to the vocal cords

Oesophagus

Common Symptoms

Difficulties in swallowing

Weight loss

Diagnostic Clues

Epidemiology

Increased risk: High intake of alcohol
All forms of tobacco use

Follow-up

By Referral to Specialist

If difficulties in swallowing: surgeon or otorhinolaryngologist as soon as soon as possible; X-ray/endoscopy

Stomach

Common Symptoms

Epigastric pain

Haematemesis/melena

Anorexia/weight loss

Difficulties in swallowing

Note: The dyspepsia may be acid

Age-distributed positive predictive value (PPV) and likelihood ratio (LR) of the cancer warning signal "Indigestion or change in bowel habits not rapidly normalized" (I) in relation to stomach cancer (StC) in general practice. (Based on a Norwegian study: see Introduction)

Age group	$P(\text{StC} \mid \text{I})$		LR	
	Males	Females	Males	Females
20–29	–	–	–	–
30–39	<0.1%	0.1%	25	27
40–49	0.3%	0.2%	23	25
50–59	1.2%	0.5%	35	29
60–69	1.3%	0.5%	15	16
70+	1.9%	1.8%	9	18

PPV = $P(\text{StC} \mid \text{I})$, probability of StC given I
Sensitivity of I presented at a consultation ($P(\text{I} \mid \text{StC})$) = 0.35

Diagnostic Clues

Epidemiology

Increased risk: Previous gastrectomy
Achlorhydria/gastritis
Nutritional factors — high intake of nitrosamines, salt and smoked food, low intake of fresh vegetables — may be associated with intestinal type (see Anatomopathology)

Medical History

Opinions differ as to whether gastrointestinal symptoms occur in "early" stomach cancer, i.e. cancer which is localized to the mucosa and submucosa and is prognostically favourable. Probably many patients experience symptoms already at this stage. (For an estimate of the sensitivity used in the table on page 30, see Introduction and its references [13, 14])

Supplementary Tests and Examinations

Occult blood in stool. In a prospective study from general practice three out of five patients with upper gastrointestinal cancer had a positive tetramethylbenzidine test (see Colon)

Iron deficiency may be present when there has been prolonged occult bleeding

Anatomopathology

- Intestinal (epidemic) type: The most frequent. Continuous formations of glandular elements. Probably dependent on nutritional factors (see Epidemiology). Decreasing incidence in the Western world
- Diffuse type: Approximately one in three cases. Poorly outlined cells infiltrating and thickening the ventricular wall. Prognosis is poor

Apudomas — rare in the stomach (see Pancreas)

Follow-up

By the General Practitioner

Practically always for dyspeptic patients who are not referred to a specialist

Always after an X-ray of the stomach ordered by the GP

If symptoms persist after negative gastroscopy, consider a double constrast X-ray to reveal/exclude a scirrhous carcinoma. Referral for another gastroscopy after a few weeks is an alternative

By Referral to Specialist

If duration of epigastric pain > 2–3 weeks: gastroscopy

In patients < 40 years of age with acid dyspepsia, an X-ray may be ordered first

After gastric resection a gastroscopy should be performed every 4–5 years, starting 10 years after an operation for gastric ulcer, 20 years after an operation for duodenal ulcer

Duodenum and Small Intestine

Common Symptoms

Abdominal pain

Diarrhoea

Bleeding, most often occult

Weight loss

Flushing (carcinoid tumours only, and usually only if they have metastasized to the liver)

Diagnostic Clues

Epidemiology

Tumours of the small intestine account for 2% of gastrointestinal tumours. About half are malignant

Carcinoid tumours are rare, like other apudomas (see Pancreas); however, after the appendix, the small intestine is the most frequent location for carcinoids

Clinical Examination

Tumours of the small intestine are occasionally palpable

Supplementary Tests and Examinations

Occult blood in stool

Iron deficiency may be present when there has been prolonged occult bleeding

Anatomopathology

Adenocarcinomas,* lymphomas and carcinoids are the most common forms

Follow-up

By Referral to Specialist

If symptoms persist after negative endoscopic and/or radiological examinations of stomach and colon, particularly if there is occult bleeding with or without iron deficiency

Colon/Rectum

Common symptoms

Change in bowel habits, e. g. constipation, diarrhoea, (most frequent for rectal tumors, thereafter tumours in the left half of the colon)

Rectal bleeding (most frequent for rectal tumours, thereafter tumours in the left half of the colon)

Mucus from the rectum

Anaemia (most frequent for tumours in the right half of the colon)

Subacute/acute obstruction developing into ileus or perforation, sometimes with a prolonged course over several days

Age-distributed positive predictive value (PPV) and likelihood ratio (LR) of the cancer warning signal "Indigestion or change in bowel habits not rapidly normalized" (I) in relation to colorectal cancer (CC) in general practice. (Based on a Norwegian study; see Introduction)

Age group	$P(CC \mid I)$ Males	Females	LR Males	Females
20 − 29	< 0.1%	−	27	−
30 − 39	0.1%	0.1%	25	27
40 − 49	0.5%	0.5%	23	25
50 − 59	2.2%	1.8%	36	30
60 − 69	2.3%	2.2%	16	16
70 +	3.4%	4.8%	9	18

PPV = $P(CC \mid I)$, probability of CC given I
Sensitivity of I presented at a consultation $(P(I \mid CC)) = 0.35$

Diagnostic Clues

Epidemiology

Increased risk: Family history of polyposis (very high risk)
                   Ulcerative colitis (highest when total colitis and
                   young age at first symptoms)
                   Previous removal of polyp
                   Probable association with high fat/low fibre diet
                   Association between alcohol and cancer of the
                   sigmoid colon shown in Japan

Increasing incidence in Western countries. Two-thirds of the cancers are located in the left half of the colon, but a greater proportion of cancers and polyps are located in the right half now than a few decades ago

Clinical Examination

15%–25% of all colorectal tumours and 30%–35% of malignant colorectal tumours are < 10 cm from the anus: *digital examination* indicated
40%–45% of colorectal tumours are < 18 cm from the anus: *rectoscopy* indicated
Almost 60% of colorectal tumours are < 30 cm from the anus

Interested GPs may buy and learn to use the 30-cm flexible sigmoidoscope. However, use of the rigid 25-cm rectoscope is cheap and easy to learn and should come into common use on wide indications. The modern version uses disposable plastic tubes. Visualization beyond the rectosigmoid junction up to 18–20 cm may be considered satisfactory in general practice. The lumen must be kept in view as the scope is advanced. Do the examination as the scope is being withdrawn. Since the procedure is invasive, the informed consent of the patient is needed.

Always perform an abdominal examination including rectal digital examination before X-ray of colon or other referral.
Technique at rectal examination is important. The total mucosal circumference must be palpated. The examination is less uncom-

fortable and the conclusions are more trustworthy if the patient stands on the floor bent forward, the elbows resting on a couch, or relaxes in a gynaecological chair.

It is quite common to perform rectal examination with the patient in the supine on a flat bench with hips and knees flexed. This method may be satisfactory when the purpose is to establish whether a patient with abdominal pain has a pelvic inflammation, but usually gives an incomplete picture of the prostate and the rectal mucous membrane.

With rectal examination there should be simultaneous palpation of the pelvic abdomen.

With rectal cancer, findings at rectal examinations vary. A hard, elevated rim with a softer area proximal to the rim is not uncommon. Small cancers may not be felt even on thorough examination. It is therefore a good idea to repeat the examination after an inverval of a few weeks if symptoms persist

Emptying for rectoscopy, and position of the patient: Rectoscopy may be attempted at the first consultation without prior emptying of the bowel if the patient has defecated since breakfast. If emptying is necessary, a small-volume laxative per rectum after breakfast at home or at the toilet of the doctor's office is usually satisfactory. The position of the patient is a matter of what the doctor is used to. Knee-elbow support on a gynaecological bench is quite practical. Older patients should be supported by an attending nurse

Supplementary Tests and Examinations

Blood in stools:

— Physiological excretion: 1–3 ml/24 h
— Melena: > 50 ml/24 h
— Tumours: 2–5 ml or more per 24 hours

Malignant tumours often bleed more than polyps, but there is considerable overlap both for malignant/benign tumours and tumours/normal physiological excretion

Tests for Occult Blood

Principle: Pseudoperoxidase activity of haemoglobin causes oxidation of an uncoloured chemical compound (tetramethylbenzidine, guajac, etc.) into a coloured compound

Use: Should be used on wide indications. Most tests are sufficiently specific to necessitate follow-up of a positive test, but not sensitive enough to exclude cancer if the test result is negative. Follow-up may be guided by the sex- and age-distributed probabilities shown in the table. Bleeding is usually intermittent, so one stool sample is not enough. Three samples on different days are usually required

Diet: Necessary for at least 3 days before and during stool sampling:

— Avoid meat and food made with animal blood: the tests are not specific for human haemoglobin.
— Avoid raw vegetables and fruit: peroxidase activity, and vitamin C which may reduce test sensitivity.
— Avoid salicylates and antiphlogistic drugs: these are promotors of gastrointestinal bleeding.
— Eat food rich in fibre and residues: these stimulate bleeding from existing mucosal pathological processes.

Probability of colorectal cancer (CC) in a patient presenting the cancer warning signal "Indigestion or change in bowel habits not rapidly normalized" (I) when a test for occult blood in stool has been properly performed. (Based on a Norwegian study; see Introduction)

Age group	$P(CC \mid I$ and OBS$+)$		$P(CC \mid I$ and OBS$-)$	
	Males	Females	Males	Females
20–29	—	—	—	—
30–39	0.7%	0.7%	—	—
40–49	3.3%	3.3%	0.1%	0.1%
50–59	13.3%	10.6%	0.5%	0.5%
60–69	13.3%	13.3%	0.6%	0.5%
70+	18.9%	25.0%	0.8%	1.2%

OBS+, occult blood found in stool

OBS–, no occult blood found in stool

$P(CC \mid I)$, probability of CC given I

Calculations based on test sensitivity 80%, specificity 88%, and on prior probabilities (see Table p. 35)

Follow-up

By the General Practitioner

Always when an X-ray of colon has been ordered

Always if proctitis is diagnosed. Continue check-ups until rectoscopy negative and no rectal bleeding

By Referral to Specialist

Change in bowel habits lasting >2 weeks or overt or occult bleeding of uncertain origin in adults: X-ray of colon with double contrast images or a coloscopy should be ordered. Both examinations demand time and skill. Capacity problems may therefore necessitate initial ordering of an "ordinary" X-ray of the colon, but sensitivity for cancer as well as for polyps is unsatisfactory

High risk groups should have regular coloscopy according to a planned programme

Liver and Intrahepatic Bile Ducts

Common Symptoms

Tiredness

Weight loss

Epigastric pain

Hepatomegaly

Jaundice

Diagnostic Clues

Epidemiology

Metastases are much more frequent than primary liver cancer

Increased risk of primary hepatomas:
— Carriers of hepatitis B surface antigen ($HB_s Ag$), especially
  with simultaneous hepatitis B_e antibody
— Cirrhosis

Medical History/Clinical Examination

Increasing abdominal circumference?

Supplementary Tests and Examinations

Alkaline phosphatase almost always increased

Anatomopathology

Adults: Hepatocellular carcinomas dominate
Children: Mostly hepatoblastomas

Follow-up

By the General Practitioner

Always after ultrasound of liver/gallbladder if no other referral

By Referral to Specialist

If hepatomegaly or jaundice: surgeon or specialist in internal medicine as soon as possible
$HB_s Ag$ carriers should be followed up by a specialist in internal medicine

Gallbladder and Extrahepatic Bile Ducts

Common Symptoms

Jaundice (but usually this is preceded by other symptoms)

Persistent pain in the right hypochondrium or more uncharacteristic abdominal pain

Weight loss

Diagnostic Clues

Epidemioloy

Increased risk: Gallstones (present in more than half of patients
with cancer in gallbladder or bile ducts)
Present or previous cholecystitis

Medical History

Imitates benign gallbladder disease, but sometimes perhaps more constant and persistent symptoms. The diagnosis quite often comes as a surprise at operation. If an operation is planned it should not be postponed for long

Supplementary Tests and Examinations

Ultrasound is the primary examination method when gallbladder disease is suspected

Follow-up

By Referral to Specialist

Signs of obstructed (dilated) bile ducts on ultrasound examination require further specialist investigation

Pancreas

Common Symptoms

Weight loss

Pain, not very intense, but persistent

Jaundice if the head of pancreas is involved

Diagnostic Clues

Epidemiology

Increased risk: High intake of alcohol
                  Cigarette smoking

Incidence ratio males : females is approximately 2 : 1

Pancreas is the most frequent location of many of the rare apudomas originating in neuroendocrine cells. Many of these apudomas are malignant. Their secretions rather than their size dominate the clinical picture. Gastrinomas and insulinomas are the least rare forms

Medical History/Clinical Examination

Vague but persistent and progressing abdominal symptoms plus weight loss should suggest the possibility of pancreatic cancer

Rarely, a new case of diabetes may signal pancreatic cancer. Around the age of 50–60 years diabetes is less common and may justify ultrasound or other examination of the pancreas

Supplementary Tests and Examinations

Ultrasound is the primary examination method when pancreatic cancer is suspected

The sedimentation rate is often high — possibly due to advanced disease at diagnosis?

Follow-up

By Referral to Specialist

The sensitivity of ultrasound varies from 60%–100% in different studies. Many supplementary specialist investigations are available, and symptoms may justify referral even when ultrasound gives negative results

Nasal Cavities and Accessory Sinuses

Common Symptoms

Persistent unilateral purulent rhinitis

Repeated unilateral nose bleeding

Nasal stenosis

Pain

Symptoms arising from pressure on adjacent structures: teeth, lacrimal duct, orbit

Diagnostic Clues

Clinical Examination

Anterior rhinoscopy: Sore/polyp with a rugged surface

Inspection/palpation of palate

Transparency of accessory sinuses may be evaluated with a special lamp

Follow-up

By Referral to Specialist

Polyp, recurrent sinusitis or persistent unilateral nose symptoms: otorhinolaryngologist

Larynx

Common Symptoms

Hoarseness > 1 week

A sensation of lump in the throat

Blood-tinged expectorate

Diagnostic Clues

Epidemiology

Increased risk: Smoking
                  High intake of alcohol

Clinical Examination

There are wide indications for inspection of the larynx. Indirect
laryngoscopy may be difficult for general practitioners without
daily practice. Right-angle telescopic laryngoscopy gives consid-
erably simpler visualization of the larynx as well as of the hypo-
pharynx and the nasopharynx. Indirect laryngoscopy with a
distal light is second-best and cheap. Anti-dew liquid may replace
warming the mirror in an alcohol flame

A supraglottic tumour may cause a lump sensation to precede
hoarseness

Follow-up

By the General Practitioner

Hoarseness < 1 month in adults > 40 years of age should be followed until a cure if an infectious agent is suspected of causing
the hoarseness

By Referral to Specialist

Any nodes on the vocal cords, duration of symptoms > 1 month,
or incomplete visualization of vocal cords: otorhinolaryngologist

Trachea, Bronchus and Lung

Common Symptoms

Cough > 1 month (in about one case in two) or, in cases of chronic cough, a change in coughing pattern

Dyspnoea (in about one case in three)

Haemoptysis (in about one case in four)

Thoracic pain (in about one case in four)

Recurrent infection of lower respiratory tract (in about one case in four)

Paraneoplasias may occur. Polyneuritis/endocrinopathy are the least rare manifestations

Age-distributed positive predictive value (PPV) and likelihood ratio (LR) of "Hoarseness or coughing without any apparent reason" (C, H) in relation to cancer or trachea/bronchus/lung (LC) in general practice. (Based on a Norwegian study; see Introduction)

Age group	$P(LC \mid C, H)$		LR	
	Males	Females	Males	Females
20–29	–	–	–	–
30–39	–	0.1%	–	42
40–49	–	0.2%	–	36
50–59	–	0.8%	–	28
60–69	6.4%	0.8%	38	21
70+	–	1.1%	–	25

PPV = $P(LC \mid C, H)$, probability of LC given C, H

Sensitivity of C, H presented at a consultation ($P(C, H \mid LC)$) = 0.25

Diagnostic Clues

Epidemiology

Increased risk: Cigarette smoking
                   Professional exposure to various kinds of dust
                   Chronic obstructive bronchitis
                   Low intake of vitamin A (vegetables, milk)

Revision of probability of lung cancer (LC) in a patient presenting "Hoarseness or coughing without any apparent reason" (C, H) in general practice, taking account of smoking habits in the age group 60–69 years

	Males	Females
$P(LC \mid C, H)$	6.4%	0.8%
$P(LC \mid C, H$ and DS)	8.5%	2.0%
$P(LC \mid C, H$ and no DS)	3.3%	0.3%

DS, daily smoking; for other abbreviations and probabilities see previous table
Sensitivity of DS 60–69 years = 80% (males), 70% (females)
Frequency of DS in general population 60–69 years = 40% (males), 23% (females)
Frequency of DS in coughers 60–69 years = 60% (males), 30% (females)

Medical History

Risk factors should be noted

If the patient presents one of the common symptoms listed, ask about the others

Haemoptysis is a scaring symptom which quite often is not reported spontaneously by the patient

Clinical Examination

Operable cases are quite often discovered on routine X-ray examination of lungs. A good medical history and an active attitude to follow-up of smokers with infections in the lower respiratory tract may improve clinical detection

Inspection of thorax/collum, percussion and auscultation may give clinical clues depending on the location of the tumour: central (most frequent), peripheral (frequently symptomless in earlier stages), mediastinal spread

Supplementary Tests and Examinations

Order an X-ray in 4–6 weeks when antibiotics are prescribed for lower respiratory tract infection in a smoker > 40 years old

If coughing is productive it is possible to send the expectorate for a cytological examination while waiting for the X-ray: Forceful productive morning cough, expectorate directly into 70% alcohol. Three specimens should be taken, on different mornings

Anatomopathology

Squamous epithelial carcinoma is the most frequent. Adenocarcinomas and small cell anaplastic carcinomas are also important. Carcinoids occur. Histological classification is difficult in many cases

Follow-up

By the General Practitioner

Patients with pneumonia may be followed up clinically after a couple of weeks; this must be decided on an individual basis

By Referral to Specialist

Haemoptysis or persisting symptoms: lung specialist, even if X-ray/laboratory tests are negative

Breast (Women and Men)

Common Symptoms

A lump

Eczema of the nipple

Retraction of nipple or skin

Secretion, sometimes blood-tinged

Age distributed positive predictive value (PPV) and likelihood ratio (LR) of lump in the breast (L_B) in relation to breast cancer (BC) in females consulting in general practice. (Based on a Norwegian study; see Introduction)

Age group	$P(BC \mid L_B)$	LR
20–29	0.3%	64
30–39	0.9%	27
40–49	2.6%	22
50–59	3.1%	24
60–69	5.3%	32
70+	39.3%	246

$PPV = P(BC \mid L_B)$, probability of BC given L_B.

Sensitivity of L_B presented at a consultation $(P(L_B \mid BC)) = 0.45$

Diagnostic Clues

Epidemiology

Increased risk:
- Previous breast cancer
- Breast cancer in mother or sister (greatest increase of risk in premenopause)
- Large body surface area (greatest increase of risk in postmenopause)
- No children or low parity
- Early menarche, late menopause and high age at last birth, except if high parity

  - Thyroxine replacement for several years
    (greatest increase of risk in nulliparae)
  - Several years of contraceptive pill use at a
    young age
  - Prolonged (> 15 years?) postmenopausal
    oestrogen replacement therapy
  - High intake of alcohol

Clinical Examination

Inspection in three planes before palpation, not forgetting the axillary tail or the axilla

About half of all malignant breast tumours are located in the upper, lateral quadrant

Small tumours more easily get "lost" in the central part of the gland; tumours in this location are often of considerable size when they are discovered

The relatively low predictive value of "lump in the breast" in younger and even in middle-aged women shows that many benign tumours and other benign changes perceived as a lump are presented to the general practitioner. This does not at all mean that such symptoms can be taken lightly. A general practitioner who palpates a lump should refer the patient. A general practitioner who cannot confirm the patient's finding of a "lump" should make a second appointment for follow-up (see Follow-up)

Follow-up

By the General Practitioners

A woman or an elderly man presenting a symptom located in the breast and who is not referred should have a follow-up consultation within 1 month, regardless of the findings of the general practitioner

A follow-up consultation may be a good time for the general practitioner to instruct women > 35 years old in monthly self-examination of the breast. In younger women such instruction is of more doubtful value except when a mother or a sister has had breast cancer; many young women worry about benign changes, which may lead to considerable mammography-/biopsy effort in these low incidence age groups

By Referral to Specialist

Palpable lump: *always* refer to a surgeon, even if recent mammography was negative

Apart from organized mammography screening, mammography is suggested when symptoms from the breast are presented but no palpable lump is found *and* the women belongs to one of the risk groups mentioned or the symptoms persist on follow-up, even if the clinical findings are negative or uncertain

Cervix Uteri

Common Symptoms

Irregular bleeding, particularly post-coital (see table p. 59)
Vaginal discharge, often blood-tinged, sometimes foul-smelling

Diagnostic Clues

Epidemiology

Increased risk: High parity
                       Early start of active sexual life
                       Many sexual partners
                       Several years of contraceptive pill use
                       Heavy smoking
Penile hygiene may influence incidence of cervical cancer in women

Clinical Examination

Dysplasia or cancer in situ usually give no symptoms. Symptoms at later stages depend on growth pattern. Ectocervical growth is most frequent and may give symptoms as described above. Endocervical cancer remains silent longer

General practitioners have an important role in motivating women to regular screening. When screening is centrally organized, motivation is particularly important in relation to women in risk groups who do not respond to screening programme invitations

Condyloma of cervix should have the same close follow-up as dysplasia

Supplementary Tests and Examinations

Technique at taking cervical smears is important. Cells from the transformation zone and from the cylindrical epithelium of the endocervix should be included, because the cell changes start at the transformation zone. To obtain good endocervical smears an endocervical brush is better than a spatula. Use the spatula on the whole ectocervical circumference, smear on one half of the slide, then get the endocervical material and smear it on the other half of the slide marked to identify the patient. The vaginal fornix is less important. Carry out fixation immediately

If screening is not centrally organized, the following screening routines are suggested:

- First smear around age 25 if there has been no previous pregnancy-related smear
- Second smear 1 year after the first
- Further smears every 3 years until two smears have been performed after the age of 60 years
- In older women > 65 years of age, a routine smear is justified if less than two smears have been performed after the patient reached the age of 60 years

Apart from screening routines, a smear is justified in cases of:

- Unusual irregular bleeding
- Macroscopic cervical changes
- Post-partum check-ups
- Abortion applicants

Anatomopathology

Squamous cell carcinoma with ectocervical growth is most frequent (about 90%)
Endocervical tumours are frequently adenocarcinomas

Follow-up

Referral to Specialist

Positive cytology, cervical condyloma, post-coital bleeding, unusual-looking cervix: gynaecologist

Corpus Uteri

Common Symptoms

Irregular bleeding:

- *Before* the climacteric, rarely cancer of the corpus
- *During* the climacteric, sometimes cancer of the corpus
- *After* the climacteric, cancer of the corpus until proved otherwise

(See Table p. 59)

Diagnostic Clues

Epidemiology

Increased risk: Long-term ($>$ 3–5 years) oestrogen substitution (Hormonal treatment with combinations of oestrogen/progestagen probably does not increase risk and should be preferred to oestrogen alone in women with an intact uterus. However, combined treatment may reduce the possible favourable effect of oestrogen alone on arterial disease risk. Prolonged combination therapy does not reduce and may possibly increase breast cancer risk)
Overweight (adipose women have increased oestrogenic stimulation from fat tissue and converted adrenal hormones)
No children or low parity
Early menarche, late menopause and high age at last birth, except if high parity

Supplementary Tests and Examinations

Cytological examination of the endometrium is suggested in general practice for:

— First irregular bleeding in women > 40 years of age and up to the menopause
— Post-menopausal bleeding while waiting for a specialist consultation — always refer in this age group
— Post-menopausal women belonging to one of the risk groups. In the case of prolonged oestrogen substitution, yearly cytological examination may be justified until the treatment is stopped. Five-yearly intervals in adipose or low-parity women between 50 and 70 years of age may be considered

Cervical cytology is almost always negative in cancer of the corpus

Follow-up

By the General Practitioner

Irregular bleeding pre-menopausally and a negative gynaecological examination necessitate a follow-up appointment in 2–3 months with the bleeding periods noted. If bleeding quickly becomes regular, and especially if endometrial cytology is negative as well, the probability of cancer of the corpus is very small

By Referral to Specialist

Any post-menopausal bleeding, even if a gynaecological examination points to possible bleeding from atrophic mucosa, and even if endometrial cytology is negative: gynaecologist

Repeated irregular bleeding pre-menopausally

Placenta (Choriocarcinoma)

Common Symptoms

Bleeding > 2 weeks post-partum or after a spontaneous abortion

Diagnostic Clues

Epidemiology

About half of the cases are preceded by a hydatidiform mole

Clinical Examination

A hydatidiform mole may be suspected when a "pregnant" uterus is growing faster than expected, judged by routine measurements of the distance between the symphysis and the fundus or by gynaecological examination, or when growth is normal but there is repeated vaginal bleeding

Supplementary Tests and Examinations

A human chorionic gonadotropin (hCG) pregnancy test

Follow-up

By Referral to Specialist

Persistent bleeding > 2–3 weeks, regardless of whether or not pregnancy has been suspected or confirmed in the preceding weeks

Ovary, Tube and Broad Ligament

Common Symptoms

Often relatively "silent" because moderate growth does not interfere with adjacent organs

A feeling of fullness in the pelvic region

Pain on sexual intercourse

Infrequently: irregular vaginal bleeding, due to metastasis or hormonal effect (see table p. 59)

Diagnostic Clues

Epidemiology

Increased risk: Nulliparae/low parity

The highest incidence rates are in old age, but cases occur in all age groups, even in children and young girls

Medical History/Clinical Examination

Abacterical pollakisuria or finger-thin stools may suggest pressure against the bladder or rectum

Some ovarian tumours have endocrinological activity. If so, oestrogenic activity is most common, while androgens or progesterone may be involved. Be suspicious if oestrogenic stimulation is reported in a cytological smear from a post-menopausal women

The habit of a yearly gynaecological examination should not stop at menopause

Palpation of inguinal glands should be part of the gynaecological examination

Ascites may occur

Follow-up

By the General Practitioner

Faecal matter sometimes may imitate pelvic tumours. If the general practitioner is uncertain, a follow-up appointment a few days later may clarify

By Referral to Specialist

Enlarged ovary or other tumour in the pelvic region: gynaecologist

Age-distributed positive predictive value (PPV) and likelihood ratio (LR) of genital bleeding (B_G) in relation to internal genital cancer (GC) in females consulting in general practice. (Based on a Norwegian study; see Introduction)

Age group	$P(GC \mid B_G)$	LR
20 – 29	0.1%	11
30 – 39	0.3%	8
40 – 49	0.7%	10
50 – 59	32.0%	359
60 – 69	36.0%	393
70 +	10.7%	93

PPV = $P(GC \mid B_G)$, probability of GC given B_G
Sensitivity of B_G presented at a consultation ($P(B_G \mid GC)$)

Cervical cancer:	age 20 – 39, 0.15
	age 40 – 49, 0.20
	age 50 – 59, 0.25
	age 60 + 0.30
Cancer of corpus uteri:	0.45
Cancer of ovary/tube/broad ligament:	0.05

Vulva

Common Symptoms

A sore or a lump
Eczema or leukoplakia may precede

Diagnostic Clues

Clinical Examination

Quite often older women are reluctant to ask for a gynaecological examination. Suggest a gynaecological examination if the patient hints that something is wrong "down there"

Very rarely, a swelling in Bartholin's gland may be caused by cancer. Slow healing or quick recurrence of "cyst" after surgical treatment may suggest such a possibility

Vagina

Common Symptoms

Post-coital bleeding

Vaginal discharge

Diagnostic Clues

Clinical Examination

Inspection of the vaginal wall is part of the gynaecological examination

Red, elevated, velvet-like areas may be vaginal adenosis which may precede cancer

Prostate

Common Symptoms

Most often asymptomatic for a long time

First symptom commonly from metastases, especially in the vertebral column

Symptoms which mimic adenoma of the prostate: hesitation, frequency, or low pressure of micturition; retention of urine

Dysuria/haematuria may be an early symptom if the tumour is located ventrolaterally

Diagnostic Clues

Epidemiology

The most common tumour in males

Clinical Examination

Malignant growth starts subcapsularly, usually in a dorsal position, so that a lump becomes palpable per rectum. In the more rare ventrolateral location (about one case in four), or in case of more advanced growth, the whole prostatic lobe becomes hard rather than firm on palpation

No good single screening method exists. However, because the tumour is common and possibilities for treatment are improving, case-finding may be rewarding in general practice. Any rectal examination in adult men should include a prostatic evaluation, whatever the reason for doing the examination. In old men such an examination may be offered every 2 or 3 years regardless of the reason for the consultation

Supplementary Tests and Examinations

Acid/prostatic acid phosphatase usually increases when the capsule is infiltrated by the tumour, but not usually in the early stages of growth. If the blood test is performed after vigorous palpation of the gland, false high levels may be found; it is better to postpone the blood test for a day

Alkaline phosphatase may increase because of metastases. The sedimentation rate may also be increased

Interested general practitioners may learn how to perform a biopsy for cytological evaluation using the Frantzén needle

Anatomopathology

Cytological evaluation has a sensitivity of 90%–95%, almost as good as the "gold-standard" histological examination. It is important to make a diagnosis because of the possibility of subsequent histological grading: Palpation alone cannot distinguish slow-growing cancers from aggressive cancers which should be actively treated:

- Highly differentiated tumours usually grow slowly and are present in about half of all males > 70 years of age
- Poorly differentiated tumours are often invasive and metastasizing. More active treatment is usually indicated

Follow-up

By Referral to Specialist

Always upon finding a hard lump or lobe, because of the importance of histological grading

Staging also influences treatment, not only grading. This means that if the general practitioner takes a biopsy, all positive findings should be referred to a urologist

Testis

Common Symptoms

A lump

Diffuse enlargement of one testicle

Relatively symptom-poor epididymitis

Newly acquired hydrocele in younger males

Gynaecomasty in young males

Metastases may give rise to symptoms before the primary tumour (vertebral column, lung, supraclavicular fossa, mediastinum, abdomen)

Diagnostic Clues

Epidemiology
Increased risk: Undescended testicles
                   Infertility

Depending on referral habits, about one in five patients referred for a scrotal lump has a malignant tumour of the testis. Intra-testicular benign neoplasia is much less frequent than malignant neoplasia

About 60% of patients with testicular cancer are young males 17–35 years old. About 40% are older

Prognosis is very good if the disease is not very advanced when correct treatment is started. This encourages a quite active diagnostic attitude

Clinical Examination

Palpation usually cannot distinguish a benign from a malignant tumour

Identify properly the testis and epididymis on each side in case of scrotal symptoms

Acquired hydrocele in young males may be emptied by puncture to obtain a better evaluation by palpation

Since metastases may give the first symptoms and cure may still be possible, palpation of testicles should be performed when there are unexplained symptoms from quite different organ systems in younger males, for instance when there is unexplained, persistent back pain

Supplementary Tests and Examinations

Microscopy of urine in cases of epididymitis. Absence of pyuria makes cancer somewhat more probable than when pyuria is present

Anatomopathology

Most malignant testicular tumours originate in germinal epithelium. Half are seminomas, half are various types of non-seminomas. Seminoma patients have a slightly higher average age

1% − 2% of testicular tumours originate in Leydig cells. Most are benign. Feminizing symptoms are possible, but rare

Follow-up

By the General Practitioner

All patients with haemospermia or testicular pain without any palpable tumour

Epididymitis which is not referred: always follow-up until cure

By Referral to Specialist

All males with a scrotal lump which is not a hydrocele, a spermatocele or acute epididymitis with unequivocal symptoms

Penis and Scrotum

Common Symptoms

A sore on the penis, usually close to the sulcus coronarius

Leukoplakia/infiltrate

Diagnostic Clues

Clinical Examination

Quite often older men are reluctant to see a doctor for their genital symptoms. Suggest a genital examination if the patient hints at a genital abnormality. The prepuce should be carefully retracted

Digression: the finding of smegma under the prepuce of young males may furnish an occasion to discuss penile hygiene and the possible relationship with cervical cancer in females

Kidney

Common Symptoms

Pain in the flank

Haematuria

Palpable tumour
(The triad pain in the flank, haematuria and palpable tumour together is rare, perhaps in one of ten patients. However, each of these three symptoms occurs in 30% − 50% patients with renal cancer)

Tiredness

Weight loss

Anaemia

First symptom in 10% − 20% is metastasis, usually in bone or lung

Diagnostic Clues

Epidemiology

Increased risk: Arterial hypertension
The incidence ratio males:females is approximately 3:2

Clinical Examination

Newly acquired or increasing varicocele of scrotum may on rare occasions be secondary to renal cancer

At mother-and-child clinics, abdominal flanks of infants and pre-school children should be palpated carefully to reveal any enlargement of a kidney

Supplementary Tests and Examinations

If there is microhaematuria without any signs of infection supplementary test are required. In general practice benign conditions are far more frequent than cancer as a cause of microhaematuria. In one prospective study with 38 patients one case of bladder cancer and no cases of renal cancer were found. If erythrocyte cylinders are demonstrated, glomerulonephritis is the most likely diagnosis. Nevertheless, such findings require a minimum investigation by cystoscopy and urography if the cause and the location of the bleeding are uncertain. Ultrasound may be ordered as well. In some cases renal angiography may be indicated without any urography, but this is a specialist decision

The varied symptomatology suggests that urinary tract symptoms are not necessary to justify urography

If haematuria persists after negative cystoscopy/urography, consider a cytological examination of the urine (may reveal cancer of the renal pelvis although the much more frequent renal cell carcinoma can rarely be detected this way: The last portion of morning urine, 10 ml added to 10 ml 50% alcohol

The sedimentation rate is high in about half the cases of renal cancer. Serum calcium may rarely be increased. Creatinine levels should be determined

Haemoglobin/haematocrit sometimes may be increased up to values suggesting (secondary) polycythaemia, but anaemia is more common

Follow-up

By the General Practitioner

Always after urography/ultrasound has been ordered

By Referral to Specialist

Urologist or surgeon can do cystoscopy/urography in one session at the same time as the indication for a retrograde examination is considered. The general practitioner therefore may choose to refer directly instead of first ordering a urography in cases of haematuria. Waiting lists and local expertise may influence the choice

When the general practitioner considers that computer tomography or angiography is indicated: urologist or surgeon

If haematuria persists after a negative minimum investigation programme, a new referral may be considered 2–3 months later

Bladder

Common Symptoms

Haematuria

Dysuria/pollakisuria is uncommon but may occur, in which case there is usually no bacterial growth

Diagnostic Clues

Epidemiology

Increased risk: Smoking
                 Certain industrial chemicals

Medical History

Occupation? Exposure to chemicals?

Supplementary Tests and Examinations

Microscopy of urine should be part of most investigations for abdominal symptoms

The haematuria may be macroscopic. In a Danish prospective multipractice study neoplasia was found in 11% of 351 general practice patients consulting for first time macroscopic haematuria. Most were bladder cancer, some were prostate, ureter or kidney cancer. Several tumours in females were located in the genital organs. It is not uncommon that vaginal or even anal bleeding is presented to the doctor as macroscopic haematuria.

Follow-up

By Referral to Specialist

Microscopic or macroscopic haematuria of uncertain origin/cause (see Kidney)

Malignant Melanoma

Common Symptoms

A mole which *grows* or which exhibits some form of *disorder:*

— Colour change over time or variation in colour (bluish/red-dish/grey-white/various shades of brown and black)
— Irregular or fading border or surface
— Ulceration/bleeding
— Asymmetry/satellites
— Loss of hair on naevus
— Hypopigmented halo if the mole is eccentric

Pigment may be absent from some melanomas, usually of nodular or acral type. These often have few and moderate symptoms: itching/erythema with or without a little lump or a sore, sometimes located where a naevus has previously disappeared

Diagnostic Clues

Epidemiology

Increased risk: Repeated exposure to intense sunshine
Sunburn, especially in blue-eyed and light-skinned persons (Sun filter creams probably protect against skin cancer)

Most malignant melanomas are new growths, but some grow from benign moles

Large congenital naevi in some cases (perhaps in about 5% — 15% of cases) may develop into malignant melanomas

Prognosis of malignant melanoma is related to the depth of its growth

Clinical Examination

Inspection should be carried out in a *sharp light* to look for variations or changes in colour. Stretching of the skin may facilitate the demonstration of pigment variation or erythema.

Lesions should be *measured* in millimeters for later comparison and before surgical removal

Localization: Depends on histological type. All parts of the body can be involved. There is an even sex distribution for face/neck. Malignant melanomas on the trunk are twice as frequent in males as in females. Malignant melanomas on the extremities are more than twice as frequent in females as in males, especially on the lower extremities, and the calves in particular

Pigment beneath the nails: Blood pigment usually has an even distribution and a sharply demarcated border parallel with the distal edge of the nail. Malignant changes are more irregular than haemorrhagic colouring, with partly merging white and pigmented streaks perpendicular to the edge of the nail

Moles which disappear are usually innocent, but the area may be watched for some months because of the rare but possible development of amelanotic melanoma (see Common Symptoms). A hypopigmented halo around a persisting or disappearing mole may be considered innocent if it is concentric. An eccentric mole in a halo should lead to referral

Anatomopathology

Pigment-forming melanocytes stem from the neural crest. Malignant melanomas may arise wherever such cells are found, but the skin is by far the most common site. They may occur in the retina and very rarely in the gastrointestinal tract or other locations

Most common: Superficial spreading melanomas (SSM). All parts of the body. Irregularities as described under Common Symptoms. There is a prolonged phase of superficial growth before deep invasion

Second most common: Nodular melanomas (NM). All parts of the body. They are protruding, sharply limited, less colourful and usually have nuances of blue–grey–black. Early lesions may be perceived by the patients as "blood blisters". Rapid deep growth

Lentigo maligna melanomas: Found on exposed surfaces, usually in older persons. Initial lesions are always flat and may resemble freckles, although the capacity to freckle disappears in early adulthood. A prolonged pre-invasive phase gives rise to coin-sized lesions. Small intralesional nodules or satellites may signal deep growth

Acral malignant melanoma: Found on the nail bed, sole and palm. Nail bed: see Clinical Examination. Moles on soles or palms should be carefully inspected and referred if there is any doubt. Both superficial and nodular types occur. The two most common locations are the heel and the nail bed of the big toe

Dysplastic naevi are probably potential precursors of malignant melanomas and may occur as an isolated condition or as part of a family syndrome. Histologically proven dysplastic moles should prompt another thorough clinical examination, removal of suspect lesions (but not of all moles on the body!), prophylactic advice and an invitation to return for consultation in the case of any subsequent mole "disorder"

Follow-up

By Referral to Specialist

Suspect lesions (see Common Symptoms) and moles with a diameter of >9 mm should be removed by a surgeon or dermatologist

Eccentric moles in a halo or moles in nail bed, palm or sole should be referred in case of any doubt

Congenital moles >1 cm in diameter may be referred before puberty if plastic surgery is considered possible. Malignancy almost never develops before puberty in such lesions

Spindle Cell and Basal Cell Carcinoma

Common Symptoms

A sore which does not heal

Small lump or wart-like lesion easily ulcerated and bleeding. Basal cell carcinomas often have a raised pearly border with a central depression

Diagnostic Clues

Epidemiology

Spindle cell carcinomas (= squamous cell carcinomas) are much less frequent, but require more active treatment than basal cell carcinomas (= basal cell epitheliomas)

Clinical Examination

Localization, spindle cell carcinomas: Face most common, often lip or auricle. External genitalia (classified as cancer of penis or vulva). Back of the hand. May also arise anywhere on the body, spontaneously or in old wounds, e.g. in scars secondary to operations/burns. Sometimes preceded by leukoplakia or by senile keratosis characterized by erythema/hyperkeratosis on atrophic skin

Localization, basal cell carcinoma: Usually exposed skin, most often the face. Probably no metastatic potential, but sometimes considerable invasive capacity

Follow-up

By Referral to Specialist

Always refer sores lasting $> 2 - 3$ months for a biopsy

Age-distributed positive predictive value (PPV) and likelihood ratio (LR) of the warning signals "Any sore which does not heal" or "Changes in colour or size of warts and moles" (S, M) in relation to skin cancer (SC), excluding basal cell carcinoma and lip cancer, in general practice. (Based on a Norwegian study; see Introduction)

| | P(SC | SM) | | LR | |
Age group	Males	Females	Males	Females
20−29	0.7%	1.5%	167	253
30−39	−	2.5%	−	128
40−49	1.8%	−	85	−
50−59	−	3.5%	−	129
60−69	2.1%	−	39	−
70+	4.2%	4.8%	37	58

PPV = P(SC | S, M), probability of SC given S, M
Sensitivity of S, M presented at a consultation (P(S, M | SC)) = 0.5

Cutaneous Paraneoplasia

Common Symptoms

Cutaneous paraneoplasias are rare, but take many forms:

- Acanthosis nigrans (axilla, groin), frequently with simulta-
  neous gastrointestinal cancer, often in stomach
- Acquired ichthyosis
- Generalized pruritus
- Erythroderma
- Purpura
- Dermatomyositis (face/eyelid: erythema/oedema/telangiectasia,
  frequently associated with cancer in female genitalia/breast
- Bowen's disease: Intraepidermal squamous cell carcinoma, cli-
  nically and histologically intermediate between senile keratosis
  and squamous cell carcinoma (see Spindle Cell and Basal Cell
  Carcinoma)

Diagnostic Clues

Epidemiology

Besides the malignancies mentioned above, lymphomas, my-
elomas, leukaemias and adenocarcinomas are the forms of cancer
most frequently associated with distant, non-metastatic (paraneo-
plastic) manifestations of the skin

Kaposi's sarcoma (multiple pigmented vascular tumours in the
dermis/epidermis uni- or bilaterally on the extremities or on the
face/neck) may occur together with other forms of cancer.
Formerly a very rare form of cancer in old people, it has become
the most important acquired immune deficiency syndrome
(AIDS) associated cancer, seen especially in male homosexuals

Herpes zoster patients do not have cancer any more frequently
than other people of the same age

Eyeball

Common Symptoms

Unilateral disturbances of vision (melanoma) depending on how close the tumour is to the macular region: a small, peripherical reduction of the field of vision is not easily noticed by the patient

A shadow in the pupil (retinoblastoma in infants)

Exophthalmus with or without periorbital haematoma (retinoblastoma, or metastasis from a neuroblastoma in children)

Diagnostic Clues

Epidemiology

In adults melanomas are the most common tumours of the eyeball

Clinical Examination

During ophthalmoscopy it is important to include examination of the periphery of the fundus

Routine red reflex examination in infants should be part of the mother-and-child clinic control programme

Neuroblastoma (originating in sympathetic nerve cells) which has metastasized to the orbit has been mistaken as a sign of child battering

Brain

Common Symptoms:

General symptoms:

- Headache (in about one case in three; in case of metastases in half of the patients)
- Nausea/vomiting (about one case in four)
- Vertigo (about one in five)
- Psychic changes/disturbances of consciousness (about one in five)

Focal symptoms, according to the localization of the tumour:

- Epilepsy (in about one case in seven or eight)
- Pareses (rare)

Special symptoms, according to the kind of tumour:
Pituitary tumour: Disturbances of vision (in more than one-half of cases). Initially these are often temporary and unilateral: after a while there is development towards bitemporal hemianopsia
Hyper-/hypopituitarism is less frequent, except with prolactinomas which are common but frequently asymptomatic
Amenorrhoea (women) or impotence (men) is sometimes a symptom of hyperprolactinemia
Acoustic neurinoma: Unilateral disturbance of hearing, unilateral noise in the ear and vertigo

Diagnostic Clues

Epidemiology

Almost 10% of brain tumours occur in children, and brain tumours constitute about 30% of all malignancies in childhood

Medical History

Any headache requires a thorough medical history to clarify location, duration, intensity, etc.

Headache mainly in the morning is suggestive of tumour, but is then usually a rather late symptom

Vertigo may be an initial symptom of fast-growing brain tumours, but in general vertigo is rarely a first symptom

Clinical Examination

Donder's test or another simple test of the visual field (pituitary tumours)

Check for nystagmus (in cases of acoustic neurinoma it is often present toward the afflicted side)

Fundal Examination

Test cranial nerves. Among possible findings is unilaterally reduced corneal reflex in acoustic neurinoma

Test tendon reflexes/motor function/sensibility/balance

Blood pressure is usually not affected

The most common primary foci of brain metastases are lung, skin (malignant melanoma), urogenital tract, breast and stomach

If headache in a child is caused by a tumour, there will usually be positive clinical findings on neurological examination including opthalmoscopy within 2−4 months

Supplementary Tests and Examinations

Serum prolactin should be measured in cases of amenorrhoea/impotence. Other hormonal analyses depend on the clinical picture

EEG: May be ordered in cases of aquired headache of uncertain origin despite a good medical history and a thorough clinical examination. The sensitivity of an EEG in relation to brain tumour has been shown in hospital studies to be quite high, around 80%. Specificity is less satisfactory, only half of 28 EEGs ordered by one Danish general practitioner in one year were normal, and none of the 28 patients had a tumour. If a slight suspicion of tumour is the only indication, repeated neurological examination or direct referral for CT of skull may be an alternative

X-ray of skull: Somewhat lower sensitivity. It may prove valuable in cases of brain tumour in children, and in cases of meningeoma, pituitary tumour, acoustic neurinoma. Visualization of sella turcica or of the internal acoustic porus may be ordered at the same time as X-ray of the skull. As usual, negative results of X-rays should be trusted less than positive clinical findings or conspicuous symptoms

CT of skull: For computerized tomography (CT), see Follow-up

Anatomopathology

Intracerebral/intramedullary: Gliomas (about 35% − 40%)
Extracerebral/extramedullary: Meningiomas (about 10%)
Pituitary tumours
(about 5% − 7%)
Acoustic neurinomas
(about 5% − 7%)
Other (about 2% − 3%): Includes medulloblastoma, a subtentorial tumour of embryonal origin, in children and young adults
Metastases (about 20% − 35%)

Follow-up

By the General Practitioner

In cases of acquired headache or vertigo which are not referred there should be a follow-up appointment in 2 − 4 weeks

By Referral to Specialist

If there is progression of symptoms or neurological findings: neurologist

If there are disturbances of vision: ophthalmologist

CT of skull should be ordered only in co-operation with a neurologist or radiologist

Spinal Cord

Common Symptoms

Pain (earliest and most frequent symptom):

- Pain in the back is often due to stretching of the periosteum and is usually most pronounced in the recumbent position
- Radiating pain is often unilateral in the cervical or lumbar part of the body and bilateral and belt-like in the thoracic part

Paresis of extremity

Loss of sensibility

Diagnostic Clues

Epidemiology

Metastases: Two to three times more frequent than primary tumors. In one hospital study, one-third of the patients with metastases had no previously known malignancy. The average age of patients with metastases is about 60 years

Primary tumours: Approximately one in three are malignant. The average age of patients with primary tumours is 35–40 years — a little lower for malignant tumours and a little higher for benign tumours

Medical History

Symptoms progress slowly in the case of primary tumours, usually for several months before the diagnosis is made

Pain aggravated by coughing, sneezing or defecation may be due to a nuclear prolapse or to a tumour in the spinal canal

Clinical Examination

The necessary examination of motor function/sensibility/tendon reflexes is the same as in any case of back pain. The patient should be examined wearing underwear only. Measurement of extremity circumference is important where there is doubt about motor function. A rectal examination should be performed, particularly if there are bilateral symptoms

Follow-up

By Referral to Specialist

If neurological findings: neurologist

Thyroid Gland

Common Symptoms

A lump

Diagnostic Clues

Epidemiology

Increased risk: Thyroid cancer in the family
High intake of the iodine in fish? (papillary form)

Incidence ratio females : males is approximately 3 : 1

Highly differentiated thyroid cancer in older people is a quite frequent finding on autopsy. Microscopically "silent" foci often remain silent, but individual cases are prognostically unpredictable

Benign tumours are five to ten times more frequent than malignant tumours

Clinical Examination

A palpable lump is the important finding and should be referred regardless of the functional status of the gland, regardless of whether the patient has a goitre, and, in a female patient, regardless of whether or not she is pregnant

Clinically it is impossible to distinguish between malignant and benign tumours, or to distinguish one malignant histological type from other types

Anatomopathology

There are four major histological types of carcinoma:

— Papillary (most frequent)
— Follicular (second most frequent)
— Medullary
— Anaplastic

Follow-up

By Referral to Specialist

If palpable lump, regardless of any result of supplementary tests like scintigraphy or thyroid function tests: surgeon

Bone

Common Symptoms

Local pain

Swelling

Diagnostic Clues

Epidemiology

Metastases are more frequent than primary tumours

A tumour in a vertebral body is usually a myeloma or a metastasis, most frequently from breast, prostate, or other parts of the urogenital tract

Medical History

Spontaneous fracture may be thought of in cases of intense, acute pain after a moderate trauma

Tumour of a vertebral body: Back pain, often slowly progressing, usually worst during the night and when the patient is lying supine. Neurological symptoms arise later on

Clinical Examination

Local pain or swelling on palpation may prompt X-ray examination of bone

Supplementary Tests and Examinations

Prolonged or unusual course of common ailments primarily thought to be tendinitis, "ordinary" back pain, coxalgia, Schlatter's disease, lesion of meniscus, etc., justifies an X-ray of the skeletal part of the region

Anatomopathology

Primary bone tumours vary from benign (osteoid osteoma) to highly malignant (osteosarcoma, Ewing's sarcoma and others). Histological classification may be difficult

Follow-up

By the General Practitioner

Acquired back pain in a patient > 40 years of age should be followed up clinically after 2–4 weeks. X-ray may be considered

Muscle and Connective Tissue

Common Symptoms

A lump or swelling

Diagnostic Clues

Epidemiology

Increased risk of sarcoma: Neurofibroadenomatosis
                              Tuberous sclerosis

All age groups

Clinical Examination

Evaluate origin and depth of infiltration when the patient tightens underlying muscles:

- Superficial tumours move freely
- A tumour infiltrating muscle will have restricted movement when muscles are tightened
- A tumour infiltrating bone will not move whether the muscles are tensed or relaxed

Soft tissue sarcomas most commonly have a deep location in or between muscles

Follow-up

By Referral to Specialist

A soft tissue tumour suspected of being malignant *must never be biopsied!* Direct referral to an oncologist or to an oncologic surgeon of:

- Any deep tumour, regardless of size
- Any subcutaneous tumour > 5 cm in diameter
- Any other soft tissue tumour where malignancy is suspected

Hodgkin's Lymphoma and Non-Hodgkin's Lymphoma

Common Symptoms

A lump (lymphadenopathy)

General symptoms:

- Fever of unknown origin
- Itching, generalized or local, sometimes intense, may come and go all of a sudden
- Night sweat
- Alcohol intolerance (pain in the thorax and the abdomen after ingestion) in some cases of Hodgkin's lymphoma (= lympho-granulomatosis)

Various focal symptoms in cases of extranodal localization, e.g. abdominal symptoms in cases of gastrointestinal lymphoma

Diagnostic Clues

Epidemiology

In young adults Hodgkin's lymphoma is more frequent than non-Hodgkin's lymphoma, but AIDS victims with non-Hodgkin's lymphoma are increasing in number. In other age groups non-Hodgkin's lymphoma is much more frequent

About 20% of malignant lymphomas start to develop extranodally, most frequently in the gastrointestinal tract

About 20% of patients with fever of unknown origin have a malignant disease

Apart from Kaposi's sarcoma, lymphomas are the most important form of AIDS-associated cancers. Their type and manifestations differ in important respects from lymphomas unrelated to HIV. Non-Hodgkin's lymphoma is by far the most frequent form even in this group of mainly young adults. Extranodal forms are more common than nodal forms. The brain and the gastrointestinal tract are the most important locations. Central nervous system lymphomas also appear to be an important complication of paediatric AIDS. Most forms are clinically aggressive, reflecting the defective immune response and immature tumour cell types. Intravenous drug abusers seem to develop AIDS-related lymphoma at least as frequently as homosexual males

Medical History

Is the patient subfebrile? In case of doubt, morning and afternoon temperatures should be measured until the next appointment

In gastrointestinal lymphoma symptoms due to tumour growth may develop more rapidly than would be expected for other forms of gastrointestinal cancer

Clinical Examination

Lymphadenopathy in general practice is very rarely due to malignant disease. A combinaton of medical history, localization, regional examination and progression or unchanged findings at the follow-up appointment must influence the decision of whether or not to refer

Inspect/palpate the drainage area of the enlarged nodes

Does the patient have hepato-/splenomegaly?

Hodgkin's lymphoma frequently starts with an isolated neck tumour. General symptoms in initial stages are more common in non-Hodgkin's lymphoma; look systematically for lymph node enlargement

Supplementary Tests and Examinations

Granulocytopenia is sometimes seen. In some cases of Hodgkin's lymphoma there is eosinophilia and/or lymphopenia

Metastases and Other Lumps in the Neck Region

Diagnostic Clues

Medical History

If regional or distant metastases are possible, take a good medical history to locate possible primary sites. The most important elements of this medical history are the natural functions and whether there have been symptoms from the oral cavity/pharynx

Clinical Examination

In one otorhinolaryngological study analyzing lumps on the upper parts of the neck, cancer was half as frequent as infection, but more frequent than developmental anomalies

Examine the adjacent drainage area: oral cavity with tongue, pharynx, tonsils. Pneumatic otoscopy may be important to reveal "silent" nasopharyngeal cancers.

For later follow-up by yourself or others: describe the tumour in relation to anatomic structures, particularly the sternocleidomastoid muscle, the thyroid gland, os hyoideum and the mandible

Anatomopathology

Malignant lumps cranically and ventrolaterally on the neck are usually metastases; lymphomas and salivary gland tumours are somewhat less frequent

Multiple Myeloma and Other Diseases Which Produce Pathological Proteins

Common Symptoms

Bone pain, most frequently in the vertebral bodies. Sometimes pathological fracture

Tiredness

Diagnostic Clues

Supplementary Tests and Examinations

Haemoglobin concentration (often low)

Sedimentation rate (often high)

Investigate proteins in serum and sometimes in urine when there is anaemia, a high sedimentation rate or persistent back pain of uncertain origin in persons > 40 years of age

Follow-up

By the General Practitioner

Acquired back pain in a patient > 40 years of age should be followed up clinically after 2 – 4 weeks. X-ray may be considered

A symptom-free patient with monoclonal gammopathy without Bence Jones proteinuria or pathological serum test results other than the gammopathy may be followed-up after a few months in general practice

By Referral to Specialist

If monoclonal gammopathy and symptoms: specialist in internal medicine

Leukaemia

Common Symptoms

Tiredness

Subfebrility

Tendency to bleeding

Lymphadenopathy

Diagnostic Clues

Medical History

Is there a history of nosebleeding or subcutaneous bleeding?

Clinical Examination

Investigate whether there is:

— Hepato-/splenomegaly
— Bleeding in the oral mucosa

Supplementary Tests and Examinations

Haemoglobin concentration, leucocyte count, blood smear and thrombocytes (at least from the blood smear) should be evaluated

In children with symptoms of uncertain origin, these tests should be carried out liberally. Sedimentation rate and C-reactive protein require vein puncture and should be investigated only when indications are somewhat stronger

Follow-up

By the General Practitioner

If general symptoms without clinical findings or pathological blood tests: follow-up appointment in 1 — 3 weeks

Polycythemia Vera

Common Symptoms

Tiredness

Various general symptoms

Diagnostic Clues

Clinical Examination

Red face/neck

75% of patients have splenomegaly, while in secondary polycythemia the spleen is usually of normal size

Supplementary Tests and Examinations

Haemoglobin concentration $> 18\,g/dl$

Sedimentation rate $0-2\,mm/h$

Haematocrit $> 55\%$

Follow-up

By Referral to Specialist

If symptoms and tests as described: specialist in internal medicine
to distinguish the primary form from polycythemia secondary to
hypoxia (erythrocytosis)

Part 3.
Frequency Tables and Flow Charts

Commentary to the Tables of Cancer Statistics

The tables presented here should give a realistic idea of which forms of cancer a general practitioner probably will have to deal with in different age groups. Nationwide statistics are presented for Scotland, England and Wales, and Canada. In the United States the National Cancer Institute runs the SEER (Surveillance, Epidemiology, and End Results) Program to identify national trends in cancer incidence and survival. Among the eleven registries participating is the State Health Registry of Iowa, whose data are presented here. Compared to other SEER areas Iowa has quite low rates of lung cancer and relatively high rates of leukaemia and non-Hodgkin's lymphoma.

All diagnoses are according to the 9th Revision of the International Classification of Diseases with its extension International Classification of Diseases for Oncology, ICD-O (WHO, Geneva, Switzerland, 1976). The tables are based on the most recent (by summer 1989) reliable registrations. The Canadian tables and the the all-ages table for England and Wales are based on 1984 figures. The other tables show annual incidence for a specified 3- to 5-year period.

ICD 9 173 (skin cancer excluding melanoma) is reported in the United Kingdom but not in Canada or the United States. Leukaemias and lymphomas are listed individually in the UK and in the US tables, while the Canadian registry has amalgamated ICD 9 200–202 (lymphomas) and ICD 9 204–207 (leukaemias). Non-Hodgkin's lymphoma is listed under ICD 9 202, lymph and histiocytic.

The percentages in the all-ages tables have a different denominator in the UK and in the American tables. For Canada and Iowa the percentages relate only to ICD 9 140–208, excluding ICD 9 173. The UK total includes ICD 9 173 as well as various in situ registrations, carcinoma in situ of the cervix being by far the most important. UK percentages would have been a little higher if the denominator had been the same as for the American percentages.

Statistics are presented by courtesy of:

Information and Statistics Division
Common Services Agency for the Scottish Health Service
Edinburgh
(Dr. J. A. Clarke and Mrs. Jan Warner)

Medical Statistics Unit
Office of Population Censuses and Surveys
London
(Mr. G. Longhorn)

National Cancer Incidence Reporting System
Health Division, Statistics Canada
Ottawa, Ontario
(Senior Analyst Leslie Gaudette)

State Health Registry of Iowa
Iowa City, Iowa
(Special Studies Coordinator Peter Weyer)

The author wishes to thank the registries and the persons mentioned for their very kind cooperation.

The ten most frequent forms of cancer in Scotland 1983 – 1986[a]
Percentage of total number of new cases and number of new cases per year

Diagnosis	Percentage	Number
Males		
Trachea, bronchus, lung	26,2	3286
Skin exluding melanoma	12,0	1511
Prostate	8,7	1096
Colon, excluding rectum	6,4	808
Bladder	6,3	793
Stomach	5,7	716
Rectum	3,9	495
Pancreas	2,5	308
Oesophagus	2,4	304
Kidney	2,0	255
Females		
Breast	17,6	2529
Skin excluding melanoma	10,3	1481
Trachea, bronchus, lung	10,1	1451
Colon, excluding rectum	7,3	1051
Stomach	3,9	565
Ovary	3,7	531
Cervix uteri	3,1	449
Rectum	3,1	440
Bladder	2,5	359
Pancreas	2,4	339

[a] Population 1983: males 2485047, females 2665358
Population 1986: males 2475039, females 2645974

The most frequent forms of cancer in **males** in Scotland 1983–1986, age distributed (the six most frequent below 55 years of age and the ten most frequent 55 years of age and older), and number of new cases per year

	Number
0–14 years	
Lymphoid leukaemia	15
Brain	14
Kidney	5
Lymph and histiocytic	5
Endocrine glands, excl. thyroid	4
Bone	4
15–29 years	
Testis	53
Hodgkin's disease	25
Brain	15
Malignant melanoma of skin	10
Lymph and histiocytic	8
Bone	7
30–54 years	
Trachea, bronchus, lung	275
Skin, excluding melanoma	205
Bladder	82
Colon, excluding rectum	82
Stomach	75
Testis	70
55–74 years	
Trachea, bronchus, lung	2106
Skin, excluding melanoma	843
Prostate	563
Bladder	477
Colon, excluding rectum	442
Stomach	425
Rectum	284
Oesophagus	189
Pancreas	178
Kidney	154

Table continued

Table continued from page 98

	Number
75+ years	
Trachea, bronchus, lung	905
Prostate	518
Skin, excluding melanoma	456
Colon, excluding rectum	279
Bladder	229
Stomach	215
Rectum	159
Pancreas	103
Oesophagus	85
Kidney	53

The most frequent forms of cancer in **females** in Scotland 1983−1986, age distributed (the six most frequent below 55 years of age and the ten most frequent 55 years of age and older), and number of new cases per year

	Number
0−14 years	
Lymphoid leukaemia	14
Brain	14
Endocrine glands, excl. thyroid	4
Kidney	3
Connective tissue, muscle	3
Lymph and histiocytic	2
15−29 years	
Cervix uteri	30
Hodgkin's disease	21
Malignant melanoma of skin	20
Breast	14
Ovary	11
Skin, excluding melanoma	10
30−54 years	
Breast	783
Cervix uteri	200
Skin, excluding melanoma	182
Trachea, bronchus, lung	144
Ovary	119
Malignant melanoma of skin	97

Table continued

Table continued from page 99

	Number
55 – 74 years	
Breast	1139
Trachea, bronchus, lung	933
Skin, excluding melanoma	643
Colon, excluding rectum	470
Ovary	283
Stomach	255
Rectum	211
Bladder	189
Body of uterus	179
Cervix uteri	168
75 + years	
Skin, excluding melanoma	646
Breast	594
Colon, excluding rectum	491
Trachea, bronchus, lung	372
Stomach	273
Rectum	188
Pancreas	152
Bladder	135
Oesophagus	122
Ovary	117

The ten most frequent forms of cancer in England and Wales 1984[a]. Percentage of total number of new cases and number of new cases

Diagnosis	Percentage	Number
Males		
Trachea, bronchus, lung	24,8	26203
Skin, excluding melanoma	11,1	11678
Prostate	9,0	9524
Bladder	6,5	6886
Stomach	6,4	6788
Colon, excluding rectum	6,3	6648
Rectum	5,0	5269
Pancreas	2,8	2926
Oesophagus	2,3	2473
Kidney	1,9	1994
Females		
Breast	19,0	21363
Skin, excluding melanoma	9,4	10576
Trachea, bronchus, lung	8,8	9840
Colon, excluding rectum	7,3	8192
Ovary	4,0	4539
Stomach	4,0	4465
Rectum	3,8	4308
Cervix uteri	3,6	4043
Body of uterus	3,0	3329
Pancreas	2,5	2772

[a] Population estimates based on 1981 census:

		Males	Females
1980	England	22638400	23828400
	Wales	1346400	1431100
1984	England	22883200	24073200
	Wales	1361000	1446200

The most frequent forms of cancer in **males** in England and Wales 1980−1984 age distributed (the six most frequent below 55 years of age and the ten most frequent 55 years of age and older), and number of new cases per year

	Number
0−14 years	
Lymphoid leukaemia	151
Brain	100
Lymph and histiocytic	41
Hodgkin's disease	37
Kidney	35
Bone	35
15−29 years	
Testis	280
Hodgkin's disease	206
Brain	98
Lymph and histiocytic	64
Bone	63
Skin, excluding melanoma	56
30−54 years	
Trachea, bronchus, lung	2116
Skin, excluding melanoma	1517
Colon, excluding rectum	675
Bladder	606
Stomach	578
Rectum	536

Table continued

Table continued from page 102

	Number
55 – 74 years	
Trachea, bronchus, lung	17493
Skin, excluding melanoma	6476
Prostate	4488
Stomach	4185
Bladder	3879
Colon, excluding rectum	3579
Rectum	3917
Pancreas	1735
Oesophagus	1396
Kidney	1118
75 + years	
Trachea, bronchus, lung	7092
Prostate	4229
Skin, excluding melanoma	3156
Stomach	2222
Colon, excluding rectum	2134
Bladder	2073
Rectum	1577
Pancreas	877
Oesophagus	652
Kidney	355

The most frequent forms of cancer in **females** in England and Wales 1980–1984 age distributed (the six most frequent below 55 years of age and the ten most frequent 55 years of age and older), and number of cases per year

	Number
0 – 14 years	
Lymphoid leukaemia	123
Brain	80
Bone	38
Kidney	30
Myeloid leukaemia	24
Connective tissue, muscle	21

Table continued

Table continued from page 103

	Number
15 – 29 years	
Cervix uteri	311
Hodgkin's disease	163
Breast	127
Malignant melanoma of skin	97
Ovary	77
Brain	73
30 – 54 years	
Breast	6172
Cervix uteri	1629
Skin, excluding melanoma	1218
Ovary	1088
Colon, excluding rectum	939
Trachea, bronchus, lung	922
55 – 74 years	
Breast	10153
Trachea, bronchus, lung	5827
Skin, excluding melanoma	4768
Colon, excluding rectum	3674
Ovary	2343
Rectum	2038
Body of uterus	2034
Stomach	1885
Cervix uteri	1641
Pancreas	1308
75 + years	
Breast	4865
Skin, excluding melanoma	4005
Colon, excluding rectum	3738
Trachea, bronchus, lung	2501
Stomach	2419
Rectum	1862
Pancreas	1278
Bladder	1049
Ovary	935
Oesophagus	844

The ten most frequent forms of cancer in Canada 1984[a]. Percentage of total number of new cases and number of new cases

Diagnosis	Percentage	Number
Males		
Trachea, bronchus, lung	21,9	9967
Prostate	16,7	7615
Colon, excluding rectum	9,2	4185
Bladder	6,7	3069
Rectum	5,0	2265
Lymphomas	4,4	1996
Stomach	4,0	1812
Leukaemias	3,0	1357
Kidney	3,0	1348
Pancreas	2,9	1304
Females		
Breast	27,1	11316
Colon, excluding rectum	10,8	4502
Trachea, bronchus, lung	8,9	3714
Body of uterus	6,2	2584
Ovary	4,5	1868
Rectum	4,2	1735
Lymphomas	4,2	1735
Cervix uteri	3,8	1576
Pancreas	2,5	1064
Bladder	2,5	1059

[a] Population estimate 1984, based on 1981 and 1986 censuses: males 12 433 500, females 12 694 400

The most frequent forms of cancer in **males** in Canada 1984, age distributed (the six most frequent below 55 years of age and the ten most frequent 55 years of age and older), and number of new cases

	Number
0 – 14 years	
Leukaemias	145
Brain	85
Lymphomas	70
Kidney	27
Endocrine glands, excl. thyroid	24
Connective tissue, muscle	17

Table continued

Table continued from page 105

	Number
15 – 29 years	
Lymphomas	206
Testis	202
Brain	91
Leukaemias	79
Malignant melanoma of skin	73
Bone	43
30 – 54 years	
Trachea, bronchus, lung	1215
Lymphomas	581
Colon, excluding rectum	496
Bladder	398
Malignant melanoma of skin	341
Rectum	311
55 – 74 years	
Trachea, bronchus, lung	6587
Prostate	4163
Colon, excluding rectum	2337
Bladder	1660
Rectum	1321
Stomach	1044
Lymphomas	849
Kidney	789
Pancreas	778
Larynx	646
75 + years	
Prostate	3288
Trachea, bronchus, lung	2153
Colon, excluding rectum	1328
Bladder	992
Rectum	624
Stomach	537
Pancreas	360
Leukaemias	314
Lymphomas	290
Kidney	258

The most frequent forms of cancer in **females** in Canada 1984, age distributed (the six most frequent below 55 years of age and the ten most frequent 55 years of age and older), and number of new cases

	Number
0 − 14 years	
Leukaemias	98
Brain	67
Lymphomas	26
Bone	25
Kidney	24
Connective tissue, muscle	23
15 − 29 years	
Cervix uteri	220
Lymphomas	191
Thyroid gland	143
Malignant melanoma of skin	111
Breast	96
Ovary	78
30 − 54 years	
Breast	3552
Cervix uteri	765
Trachea, bronchus, lung	663
Colon, excluding rectum	536
Ovary	502
Body of uterus	467
55 − 74 years	
Breast	5405
Trachea, bronchus, lung	2306
Colon, excluding rectum	2215
Body of uterus	1718
Ovary	927
Rectum	923
Lymphomas	733
Pancreas	538
Bladder	503
Stomach	452

Table continued

Table continued from page 107

	Number
75+ years	
Breast	2262
Colon, excluding rectum	1736
Trachea, bronchus, lung	737
Rectum	563
Stomach	460
Pancreas	432
Bladder	417
Body of uterus	391
Lymphomas	381
Ovary	343

The ten most frequent forms of cancer in the state of Iowa, USA, 1983 – 1985[a]. Percentage of total number of new cases and number of new cases per year

Diagnosis	Percentage	Number
Males		
Trachea, bronchus, lung	21,7	1326
Prostate	20,4	1252
Colon, excluding rectum	11,0	676
Bladder	5,2	317
Rectum	5,0	307
Lymph and histiocytic	3,6	222
Kidney	3,0	186
Pancreas	2,8	172
Larynx	2,2	137
Stomach	2,1	127
Females		
Breast	27,6	1644
Colon, excluding rectum	14,6	870
Trachea, bronchus, lung	8,1	480
Body of uterus	7,0	415
Rectum	4,5	269
Ovary	4,3	254
Lymph and histiocytic	3,7	221
Pancreas	2,8	166
Cervix uteri	2,6	154
Malignant melanoma of skin	2,0	120

[a] Total population 1980: 2913808 (census). 51% females, 49% males, 97,4% whites, 1,4% blacks, 1,2% other races
Total population 1987: 2834000 (estimate)

The most frequent forms of cancer in **males** in the state of Iowa, USA, 1983–1985, age distributed (the six most frequent below 55 years of age and the ten most frequent 55 years of age and older), and number of new cases per year

	Number
0–14 years	
Brain	11
Lymphoid leukaemia	10
Lymph and histiocytic	5
Bone	4
Endocrine glands excl. thyroid	4
Kidney	4
15–29 years	
Testis	30
Hodgkin's disease	16
Lymph and histiocytic	9
Brain	8
Malignant melanoma of skin	8
Thyroid gland	4
30–54 years	
Trachea, bronchus, lung	121
Colon, excluding rectum	59
Malignant melanoma of skin	44
Lymph and histiocytic	43
Testis	28
Rectum	28
55–74 years	
Trachea, bronchus, lung	857
Prostate	634
Colon, excluding rectum	359
Rectum	184
Bladder	174
Lymph and histiocytic	104
Kidney	98
Larnyx	96
Pancreas	84
Stomach	71

Table continued

Table continued from page 110

	Number
75+ years	
Prostate	603
Trachea, bronchus, lung	346
Colon, excluding rectum	255
Bladder	123
Rectum	96
Pancreas	61
Lymph and histiocytic	60
Kidney	58
Stomach	45
Lymphoid leukaemia	36

The most frequent forms of cancer in **females** in the state of Iowa, USA, 1983−1985, age distributed (the six most frequent below 55 years of age and the ten most frequent 55 years of age and older), and number of new cases per year

	Number
0−14 years	
Lymphoid leukaemia	9
Brain	8
Kidney	4
Connective tissue, muscle	2
Hodgkin's disease	2
Bone	2
15−29 years	
Hodgkin's disease	17
Thyroid gland	17
Malignant melanoma of skin	15
Cervix uteri	14
Ovary	7
Breast	6

Table continued

Table continued from page 103

	Number
30 – 54 years	
Breast	385
Colon, excluding rectum	71
Body of uterus	70
Cervix uteri	66
Trachea, bronchus, lung	62
Ovary	54
55 – 74 years	
Breast	775
Colon, excluding rectum	367
Trachea, bronchus, lung	308
Body of uterus	246
Ovary	125
Rectum	119
Lymph and histiocytic	100
Pancreas	67
Kidney	58
Cervix uteri	51
75 + years	
Breast	477
Colon, excluding rectum	432
Rectum	127
Trachea, bronchus, lung	109
Body of uterus	98
Lymph and histiocytic	88
Pancreas	87
Ovary	67
Bladder	61
Stomach	47

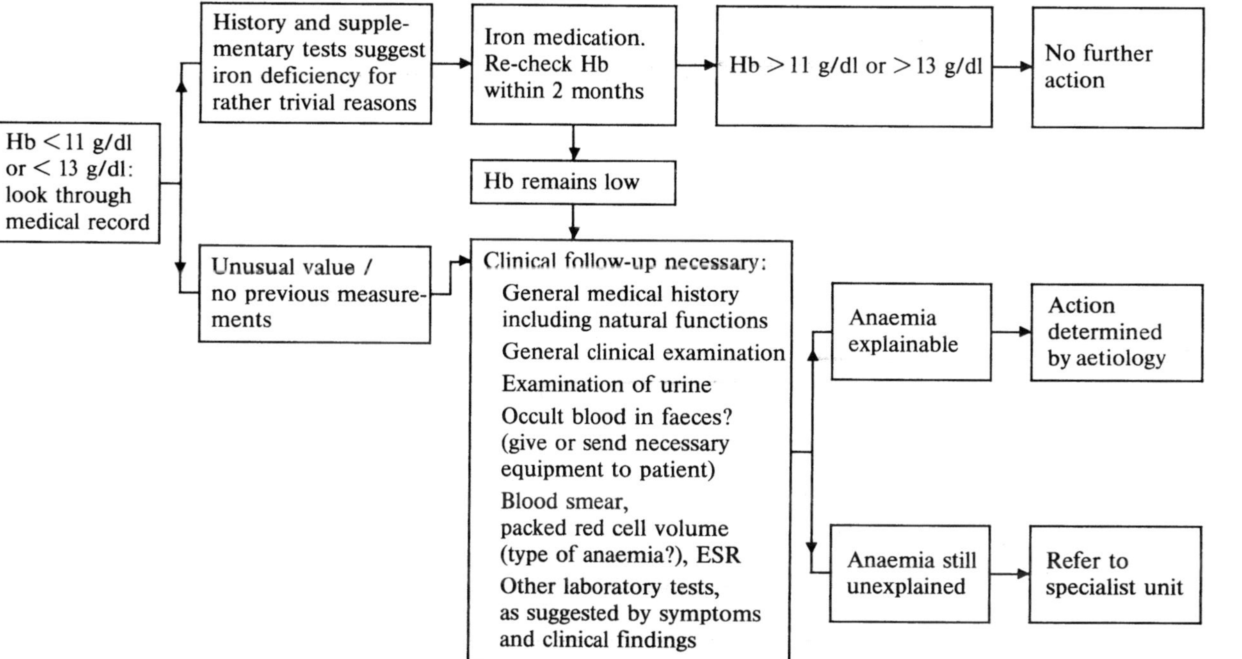

Diagnostic flow chart for patients with a measured haemoglobin concentration (*Hb*) <11 g/dl (women) and <13 g/dl (men). *ESR*, erythrocyte sedimentation rate

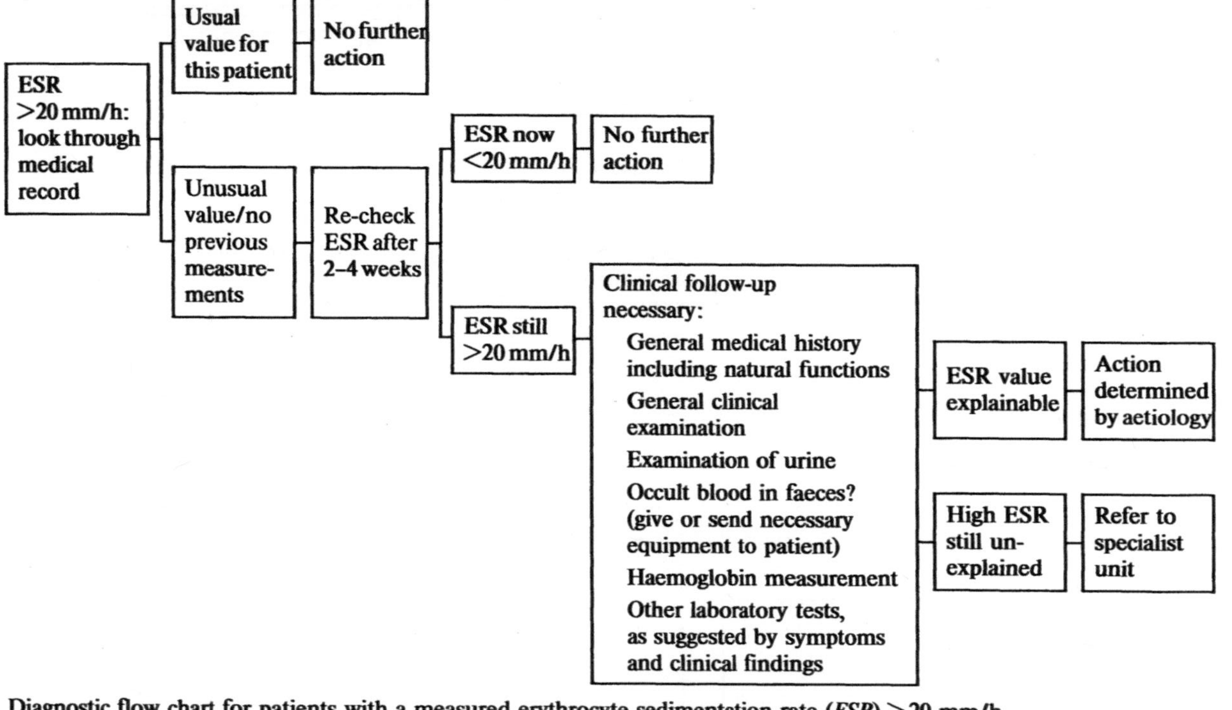

Diagnostic flow chart for patients with a measured erythrocyte sedimentation rate (*ESR*) >20 mm/h

Bibliography

Oral Cavity and Pharynx

Eneroth C-M (1971) Salivary gland tumors in the parotid gland, submandibular gland, and the palate region. Cancer 27: 1415–1418

Haugeto O, Bostad L, Solem B (1987) Svulster i glandula parotis (Tumours in the parotid gland). Tidsskr Nor Laegeforen 107: 2621–2622 (English summary)

Liavaag PG, Elgen A, Sandstad E, Lote K, Rosengren B (1989) Epipharynxcancer (Nasopharyngeal carcinoma). Tidsskr Nor Laegeforen 109: 1521–1523 (English summary)

Schrøder K, Modalsli B, Mair IWS (1977) Tumor colli. Et 5-års-materiale (Tumour colli. A five year material). Tidsskr Nor Laegeforen 97: 1434–1437 (English summary)

Skaansar K, Dahl T (1988) Pleomorft adenom i epipharynx (Pleomorphous adenoma in the epipharynx). Tidsskr Nor Laegeforen 108: 933–934 (English summary)

Digestive Organs

Bakkevold K, Pettersen A, Arnesjö B (1985) Diagnostikk ved pankreascancer (Diagnosis of pancreatic cancer). Tidsskr Nor Laegeforen 105: 2047–2049 (English summary)

Berstad T, Monclair T, Bergan A, Flatmark A (1986) Kirurgisk behandling av primær levercancer (Surgical treatment of primary liver carcinoma). Tidsskr Nor Laegeforen 106: 2140–2142 (English summary)

Berstad T, Heen L, Flatmark A, Gjone E (1988) Colitis ulcerosa og kolorektal cancer (Ulcerative colitis and colorectal cancer). Tidsskr Nor Laegeforen 108: 912–914 (English summary)

Burhol PG, Jenssen TG, Florholmen J, Jorde R (1987) Apudomer i gastrointestinaltractus og pankreas (Apudomas in the gastrointestinal tract and pancreas). Tidsskr Nor Laegeforen 107: 652–653 (English summary)

Byers T (1988) Diet and cancer. Any progress in the interim? Cancer 62: 1713–1724

Correa P, Haenszel W, Cuello C, Tannenbaum S, Archer M (1975) A model for gastric cancer epidemiology. Lancet ii: 58–59

Dybdahl JH (1984) Occult faecal blood loss determined by a ^{51}Cr method and chemical tests in patients referred for upper gastrointestinal endoscopy. Scand J Gastroenterol 19: 235–244

Dybdahl JH, Daae LNW, Larsen S (1984) Occult faecal blood loss determined by chemical tests and a ^{51}Cr method. Scand J Gastroenterol 19: 245–251

Eri LM, Hoel R (1985) Adenokarsinom i colon og rectum. En populasjonsundersøkelse (Adenocarcinoma in the colon and rectum. A population study). Tidsskr Nor Laegeforen 105: 665–668 (English summary)

Feczko PJ, Halpert RD (1986) Reassessing the role of radiology in hemoccult screening. AJR 146: 697–701

Fielding JWL, Ellis DJ, Jones BG, Paterson J, Powell DJ, Waterhouse JAH, Brookes VS (1980) Natural history of "early" gastric cancer: results of a 10-year regional survey. Br Med J 281: 965–967

Graffner H, Hallin E, Stridbeck H, Nilsson J (1986) The frequency of digital and endoscopic examination of the rectum before radiological barium enema. Scand J Prim Health Care 4: 249–251

Granlund OG (1982) Index Medicus — et forsømt diagnostikum (Index Medicus — a forgotten diagnostic aid). Tidsskr Nor Laegeforen 102: 810 (English summary)

Haug K, Schrumpf E (1985) Gastrointestinaltraktus (Gastrointestinal tract). In: Nylenna M, Gundersen S, Johannessen JV (eds) Kreft i almenpraksis (Cancer in general practice). Universitetsforlaget, Oslo (In Norwegian)

Heuch I, Kvåle G, Jacobsen BK, Bjelke E (1983) Use of alcohol, tobacco and coffee, and risk of pancreatic cancer. Br J Cancer 48: 637–643

Hirayama T (1989) Association between alcohol consumption and cancer of the sigmoid colon: Observations from a Japanese cohort study. Lancet ii: 725–727

Holliday HW, Hardcastle JD (1979) Delay in diagnosis and treatment of symptomatic colorectal cancer. Lancet i: 309–311

Jacobsen BK (1988) Grønnsaker og forebygging av kreft (Vegetables and the prevention of cancer). Tidsskr Nor Laegeforen 108: 2744–2746 (English summary)

Linnestad P, Myrvang B, Ritland S, Bergan A, Valnes K, Holst JJ (1983) Glukagonproduserende tumor i pankreas (Glukagonoma). Tidsskr Nor Laegeforen 103: 1520–1522 (English summary)

Meland E (1983) Hemofec-test — en prospectiv undersøkelse i almenpraksis (Hemofec-test — a prospective research from family practice). Tidsskr Nor Laegeforen 103: 1073–1076 (English summary)

Moland J, Danielsen S (1982) Primære tynntarmsvulster (Primary tumours of the small intestine). Tidsskr Nor Laegeforen 102: 1074–1076 (English summary)

Murakami T (1979) Early cancer of the stomach. World J Surg 3: 685–692

Øhman U (1982) Tidig ventrikelcancer — en aktuell översikt (Early cancer of the ventricle — a survey). Nord Med 97: 74–76 (English summary)

Olsen AK, Harbitz TB, Lindahl AK, Liavåg I (1986) Ulcus pepticum. Karsinom i ventrikkelen etter reseksjon (Peptic ulcer. Gastric carcinoma after resection). Tidsskr Nor Laegeforen 106: 1929–1931 (English summary)

Rosseland A, Solheim K (1983) Colorectal polyps — coloscopy. Tidsskr Nor Laegeforen 103: 1367–1368 (Editorial, in Norwegian)

Schlichting E, Buanes T, Stadaas Jo (1988) Galleveiscancer (Biliary tract cancer). Tidsskr Nor Laegeforen 108: 733–735 (English summary)

Solheim K (1987) Cancer ventriculi (Stomach cancer). Tidsskr Nor Laegeforen 107: 441–442 (Editorial, in Norwegian)

Solheim K (1988) Kolorektal cancer (Colorectal cancer). Tidsskr Nor Laegeforen 108: 903–904 (Editorial, in Norwegian)

Søndenaa K, Buanes T, Schistad P, Gerner T (1987) Maligne duodenal-tumores (Malignant duodenal tumours). Tidsskr Nor Laegeforen 107: 2630–2631 (English summary)

Winnawer SJ, Cummins R, Baldwin MP, Ptak A (1982) A new flexible sigmoidoscope for the generalist. Gastrointest Endosc 28: 233–236

Respiratory System

Geyman JP, Kirkwood R (1983) Telescopic laryngoscopy. J Fam Pract 16: 789–791

Høie J, Wium P (1985) Kreft i respirasjonsorganene (Cancer in the respiratory system). In: Nylenna M, Gundersen S, Johannessen JV (eds) Kreft i almenpraksis (Cancer in general practice). Universitetsforlaget, Oslo (In Norwegian)

Rostad H, Vale JR (1978) Primær lungecancer. En retrospektiv undersøkelse (Bronchial carcinoma). Tidsskr Nor Laegeforen 98: 1670–1673 (English summary)

Skillrud DM, Offord KP, Miller RD (1986) Higher risk of lung cancer in chronic obstructive pulmonary disease. Ann Intern Med 105: 503–507

Wist E, Melsom H, Vermund H, Winther F (1986) Behandling av avansert plateepitelcancer i maxillarsinus (Treatment of advanced squamous cell carcinoma of the maxillary sinus). Tidsskr Nor Laegeforen 106: 572–576 (English summary)

Breast and Reproductive Organs

Amlie E, Seland P, Skjørten F et al. (1987) Cancer mammae i Oslo (Breast cancer in Oslo). Tidsskr Nor Laegeforen 107: 2732–2736 (English summary)

Bergkvist L, Adami H-O, Persson I, Hoover R, Schairer C (1989) The risk of breast cancer after estrogen and estrogen-progestin replacement. N Engl J Med 321: 293–297

Bergsjø P (1981) Cytologisk endometriediagnostikk (Endometrial cytology). Tidsskr Nor Laegeforen 101: 927–928 (English summary)
Brinton LA, Schairer C, Haenszel W, Stolley P, Lehman HF, Levine R, Savitz DA (1986) Cigarette smoking and invasive cervical cancer. JAMA 255: 3265–3269
Council on Scientific Affairs (1989) Mammographic screening in asymptomatic women aged 40 years and older. JAMA 261: 2535–2542
de Waard F, Baanders-van Halewijn EA (1974) A prospective study in general practice on breast cancer risk in post-menopausal women. Int J Cancer 14: 153–160
Eyjolfson O, Jerve F (1983) Tumores i det lille bekken. Påvisning ved ultrasonografi (Tumours in the pelvic region demonstrated by ultrasonography). Tidsskr Nor Laegeforen 103: 1689–1690 (English summary)
Fosså SD et al. (1982) Svensk-norsk diagnose- og behandlingsopplegg for ikke-seminomer i testis (SWENOTECA) (The Swedish-Norwegian diagnosis and treatment program for testicular cancer). Tidsskr Nor Laegeforen 102: 371–374 (English summary)
Frank JW, Mai V (1985) Breast self-examination in young women: more harm than good? Lancet ii: 654–657
Hagen RH, Johansen TEB (1987) Benigne testistumores (Benign testicular tumors). Tidsskr Nor Laegeforen 107: 2847–2848 (English summary)
IARC working group on evaluation of cervical cancer screening programmes (1986) Screening for squamous cervical cancer: duration of low risk after negative results of cervical cytology and its implication for screening policies. Br Med J 293: 659–664
Johansen TEB, Kummen O (1987) Malignitet, fertilitet og retentio testis (Malignancy, fertility and undescended testis). Tidsskr Nor Laegeforen 107: 234–235 (English summary)
Kapdi CC, Wolfe JN (1976) Breast cancer. Relationship to thyroid supplements for hypothyroidism. JAMA 236: 1124–1127
Klepp O, Bjertnæs Aa (1985) Cancer testis. In: Nylenna M, Gundersen S, Johannessen JV (eds) Kreft i almenpraksis (Cancer in general practice). Universitetsforlaget, Oslo (In Norwegian)
Kvåle G (1989) Reproductive factors and risk of cancer of the breast and genital organs. A prospective study of Norwegian women. Thesis. Bergen, Norway: University of Bergen and the Cancer Registry of Norway
Longnecker MP, Berlin JA, Michele JO, Chalmers TC (1988) A meta-analysis of alcohol consumption in relation to risk of breast cancer. JAMA 260: 652–656
Lund E (1987) Risiko for brystkreft hos unge kvinner med mødre som har hatt brystkreft (Breast cancer in young women with a history of breast cancer in their mother). Tidsskr Nor Laegeforen 107: 12–13 (English summary)

Mack T, Casagrande JT (1981) Epidemiology of gynecologic cancer. II. Endometrium, ovary, vagina, vulva. In: Coppleson M (ed) Gynecologic oncology. Fundamental principles and clinical practice. Churchill Livingstone, Edinburgh

Mandelblatt J, Gopaul I, Wistreich M (1986) Gynecological care of elderly women. Another look at Papanicolaou smear testing. JAMA 256: 367–371

Nesheim B-I, Christoffersen T (1983) P-piller og cancer (Contraceptive pills and cancer). Tidsskr Nor Laegeforen 103: 2252–2253 (English summary)

Norwegian Department of Health and Social Welfare (1987) Mammografiscreening i Norge. Masseundersøkelse for brystkreft (Mammography screening in Norway). Universitetsforlaget, Oslo (In Norwegian; Norges Offentlige Utredninger, report no. 7)

Rekkedal OK (1986) Cancer glandula Bartholini. Tidsskr Nor Laegeforen 106: 136 (English summary)

Reichborn-Kjennerud S (1983) Condyloma acuminatum. Nye aspekter på manifestasjonsformer og betydning (Condylomata acuminata. New aspects on its manifestations and their significance. Tidsskr Nor Laegeforen 103: 1432–1435 (English summary)

Sager EM, Natvig NL, Drevvatne T (1982) Mammografi. En oversikt (Mammography. A review). Tidsskr Nor Laegeforen 102: 952–955 (English summary)

Sökeland J (1978) Cancer prostata. Hexagon 5: 18–24 (Hoffmann-La Roche; in Norwegian)

Stenehjem E, Ludvigsen TC, Rundén TØ, Waaler G, Øgreid, PI, Schei OM (1988) Digital rektal eksplorasjon som screening for cancer prostatae (Digital rectal exploration as screening for prostatic cancer). Tidsskr Nor Laegeforen 108: 674–675 (English summary)

Vaage S, Foerster A, Kirkhus B, Heilo A, Halse J, Johannesen ØM (1988) Endokrinopati og Leydig-celletumor i testis (Endocrinopathy and Leydig cell tumor i testis). Tidsskr Nor Laegeforen 108: 922–924 (English summary)

Urinary Tract

Fryjordet A, Wæhre H (1982) Perifert infiltrerende nyrebekkencancer (Flat infiltrating carcinoma of the renal pelvis). Tidsskr Nor Laegeforen 102: 428–429 (English summary)

Gravdahl HK, Grøttum K (1984) Nyrecancer i Troms 1974–1978 (Renal cancer in Troms, Norway, 1974–1978). Tidsskr Nor Laegeforen 104: 1295–1298 (English summary)

Iversen BM (1987) Asymptomatisk hematuri (Asymptomatic haematuria). Tidsskr Nor Laegeforen 107: 1251–1253 (English summary)

Otnes B, Rimstad K (1980) Utredning og kontroll ved hematuri uten sikker årsak (Control of microhaematuria of uncertain origin). Tidsskr Nor Laegeforen 100: 1762–1765 (English summary)

Ous S, Berdal S (1985) Urinveier (Urinary organs). In: Nylenna M, Gundersen S, Johannessen JV (eds) Kreft i almenpraksis (Cancer in general practice). Universitetsforlaget, Oslo (In Norwegian)

Patel NP, Lavengood RW (1978) Renal cell carcinoma: natural history and results of treatment. J Urol 119: 722–726

Pedersen C, Svendsen LB, Hvidt V, Pedersen PA (in preparation). The prognosis of macroscopic haematuria in general practice

Skinner DG, Colvin RB, Vermillion CD, Pfister RC, Leadbetter WF (1971) Diagnosis and management of renal cell carcinoma. A clinical and pathologic study of 309 cases. Cancer 28: 1165–1177

Tönies H (1986) Causes of microhaematuria in an Austrian general practice. Scand J Prim Health Care 4: 25–28

Skin

Akslen, LA, Hove LM (1987) Malignt melanom — amelanotisk type (Malignant melanoma — amelanotic type). Tidsskr Nor Laegeforen 107: 371–372 (English summary)

Day CL, Lew RA, Mihm MC, Harris MN, Kopf AW, Sober AJ, Fitzpatrick TB (1981) The natural break points for primary-tumor thickness in clinical stage I melanoma. N Engl J Med 305: 1155

Elwood FM, Gallagher RP, Hill GB, Spinelli FF, Pearson FCG, Threlfall W (1984) Pigmentation and skin reaction to sun as risk factors for cutaneous melanoma: Western Canada Melanoma Study. Br Med J 288: 99–102

Fyrand O (1978) Solbestråling og cancerutvikling i huden (Exposure to the sun and cancer development in the skin). Tidsskr Nor Laegeforen 98: 1139–1140 (English summary)

Fyrand O (1985) Dermadromer — hudens reaksjon på endel indremedisinske tilstander (Skin reactions to internal medical conditions). Farmakoterapi 41: 1–13 (In Norwegian)

Hove LM, Akslen LA (1987) Malignt melanom i hud (Malignant melanoma of the skin). Tidsskr Nor Laegeforen 107: 17–19 (English summary)

Kavli G (1983) Genitale sår (Genital ulcera). Tidsskr Nor Laegeforen 103: 1882–1884 (English summary)

Kelly JW, Crutcher WA, Sagebiel RW (1986) Clinical diagnosis of dysplastic melanocytic nevi. A clinicopathologic correlation. J Am Acad Dermatol 14: 1044–1052

Larsen TE (1988) Maligne melanomer og deres forstadier (Malignant melanomas and their percursors). Tidsskr Nor Laegeforen 108: 1398–1402 (English summary)

Mihm MC Jr, Clark WH Jr, Reed RJ (1975) The clinical diagnosis of malignant melanoma. Sem in Oncol 2: 105–118
Moan J, Volden G (1983) Er det sunt eller skadelig å sole seg? (Sunbathing – healthy or risky?). Tidsskr Nor Laegeforen 103: 1425–1429 (English summary)
Ragozzino MW, Melton LJ, Kurland LT, Chu CP, Perry HO (1982) Risk of cancer after herpes zoster. A population-based study. N Engl J Med 307: 393–397
Wist E, Solheim ØP (1984) Kaposis sarkom (Kaposi's sarcoma). Tidsskr Nor Laegeforen 104: 495–498

Eye and Central Nervous System

Erichsen GGA (1989) EEG til påvisning af primære intrakraniale svulster i almenpraksis. Anvendelsesområde og begrænsning (EEG demonstration of primary intracranial tumours, as applicable to general practice; scope and limits of its use). Nord Med 104: 69–71 (English summary)
Hanssen KF, Norman N, Nesbakken R (1982) Behandling av prolaktin-produserende hypofysetumores (Treatment of prolactin producing pituitary adenomas). Tidsskr Nor Laegeforen 102: 1222–1225 (English summary)
Honig PJ, Charney EB (1982) Children with brain tumor headaches. Am J Dis Child 136: 121–124
Segal AJ, Fishman RS (1975) Delayed diagnosis of pituitary tumors. Am J Ophthalmol 79: 77–81
Sortland O (1982) Røntgendiagnostikk ved svulster i den cerebello-pontine vinkel (Radiological diagnosis of tumours in the cerebello-pontine angle). Tidsskr Nor Laegeforen 102: 683–687 (English summary)
Todnem K, Strandjord RE, Slettebø H, Mørk SJ (1984) Intraspinale neoplasmer (Intraspinal neoplasms). Tidsskr Nor Laegeforen 104: 1528–1532 (English summary)
Unsgård G, Kufaas T, Moe PJ (1981) Aspekter ved neuroblastom (Aspects of neuroblastoma). Tidsskr Nor Laegeforen 101: 1513–1515 (English summary)
Wang M, Hatlevoll R (1986) Medulloblastom. Postoperativ behandling (Medulloblastoma. Postoperative treatment). Tidsskr Nor Laegeforen 106: 216–218 (English summary)
Watne K (1983) Intrakranielle metastaser ved cancer mammae (Intracranial metastases associated with cancer mammae). Tidsskr Nor Laegeforen 103: 2234–2236 (English summary)
Wilson J, Holmsen R (1983) Tumores i nervesystemet. Forekomst, klinikk og undersøkelsesmetoder i Akerhus fylke 1974–1978 (Tumours of the nervous system. Epidemiology, clinical presentation and methods of investigation in the Norwegian county of Akershus, 1974–1978). Tidsskr Nor Laegeforen 103: 2162–2165 (English summary)

Thyroid Gland

Solem JH, Sund T, Helsingen N, Nerdrum HJ (1984) Thyreoideascintigrafi. Den diagnostiske verdi ved utredningen av den solitære thyreoideaknute (Prediction of malignancy in solitary thyroid nodules. The value of preoperative scintigraphy in a prospective study of 202 patients). Tidsskr Nor Laegeforen104: 297−299 (English summary)
Søndenaa K, Halvorsen JF, Varhaug JE, Skarstein A, Grong K (1986) Cancer thyreoidea. Et 10-årsmateriale. (Thyroid cancer. A 10-year study). Tidsskr Nor Laegeforen 106: 2137−2139 (English summary)

Bone, Muscle and Connective Tissue

Alho A (1986) Aggressive og maligne bentumores. Konserverende radikal kirurgi (Aggressive and malignant bone tumors. Radical sparing surgery). Tidsskr Nor Laegeforen 106: 734−738 (English summary)
Solheim Ø, Stenwig AE, Talle K, Høie J (1987) Bløtvevsarkom. Prinsipper for primærdiagnostikk, utredning og behandling (Soft tissue sarcoma. The principles of diagnosis, examination and treatment). Tidsskr Nor Laegeforen 107: 255−257 (English summary)
Terjesen T (1979) Maligne vertebrale tumores (Malignant vertebral tumours). Tidsskr Nor Laegeforen 99: 1713−1715 (English summary)

Lymphatic and Haemopoietic Tissue

Aaraas I, Grøttum KA (1985) Blod- og lymfekreft (Blood and lymphatic cancer). In: Nylenna M, Gundersen S, Johannessen JV (eds) Kreft i almenpraksis (Cancer in general practice). Universitetsforlaget, Oslo (In Norwegian)
Allhiser JN, McKnight TA, Shank JC (1981) Lymphadenopathy in a family practice. J Fam Pract 12: 27−32
Bruserud Ø (1983) Feber av ukjent årsak ved maligne sjukdommar hos vaksne (Fever of unknown origin in adults with malignant disease). Tidsskr Nor Laegeforen 103: 1790−1792 (English summary)
Melsom H, Rode L, Kaalhus O, Elgjo RF, Langholm R, Marton P (1982) Non-Hodgkin lymfom lokalisert i gastrointestinaltractus (Non-Hodgkin lymphoma involving the gastrointestinal tract). Tidsskr Nor Laegeforen 102: 374−377 (English summary)